# Dental Nurse Survival Guide

**Other Quay Books titles in dental care include:**

*Professionalism and Ethics: A guide for dental care professionals*
*Continuing Professional Development: A resource for dental care professionals*
*The Dental Nurses' Guide to Infection Control and Decontamination*
*The Management of Medical Emergencies: A guide for dental care professionals*

**Series editor**
   Dr John Fowler

**Note**

*Healthcare practice and knowledge are constantly changing and developing as new research and treatments, changes in procedures, drugs and equipment become available.*

*The author and publishers have, as far as is possible, taken care to confirm that the information complies with the latest standards of practice and legislation.*

# Dental Nurse Survival Guide

*by*

**Kathryn Porter**

Quay Books Division, MA Healthcare Ltd, St Jude's Church, Dulwich Road, London SE24 0PB

British Library Cataloguing-in-Publication Data
A catalogue record is available for this book

© MA Healthcare Limited 2011

ISBN-10: 1-85642-409-X
ISBN-13: 978-1-85642-409-7

All rights reserved. No part of this publication may be reproduced, stored in a retrieval system or transmitted in any form or by any means, electronic, mechanical, photocopying, recording or otherwise, without prior permission from the publishers

Cover design by Louise Cowburn, Fonthill Creative
Associate Publisher: Thu Nguyen

Printed by CLE, Huntingdon, Cambridgeshire

# Contents

*About the author* vi
*Introduction* vii

## Section 1: Clinical Practice

**Chapter 1:** *Dealing with medical emergencies* — 1

**Chapter 2:** *Dealing with dental emergencies* — 19

**Chapter 3:** *Dealing with daily practice* — 25

**Chapter 4:** *Preventing cross infection* — 37

**Chapter 5:** *Radiology* — 51

**Chapter 6:** *Role in the care of patients during treatment* — 61

**Chapter 7:** *Role in telling patients bad news* — 83

## Section 2: Professional Practice

**Chapter 8:** *Professional practice requirements and CPD* — 87

**Chapter 9:** *The dental practice team and culture* — 105

*Index* — 111

# About the author

Kathryn (Kathy) Porter recently retired from dental nursing in 2011, having started her training in September 1968 at Birmingham Dental Hospital and qualifying in 1970. Apart from a short time working in the dental department of a large industrial complex, she has worked at Birmingham Dental Hospital until her retirement. She was appointed Senior Dental Nurse in 1973 and promoted to Assistant Principal Dental Nurse in 1989. In 2007 her job title changed to Senior Dental Nurse (Decontamination).

Kathy trained as an Infection Control Link Nurse, now known as Infection Prevention and Control Link Practitioner, in 2003 and this began her keen interest in infection control and decontamination good practice. After being invited to sit on the Editorial Board of *Dental Nursing* in 2005, Kathy began to write articles on the subject of infection prevention and control and was also invited to write a book *The Dental Nurses' Guide to Infection Control and Decontamination* which was published in 2008. Although published before the notorious *Health Technical Memorandum 01-05*, her book proposes the same, and even higher standards, than those outlined in the HTM 01-05 document, and has become recommended for all dental nurses and dental care professionals (DCPs) as a point of reference on the topic. Kathy has given talks on the subject in various venues to provide verifiable continuing professional development for all DCPs.

Kathy intends to enjoy her retirement, pursuing her interests in travelling, watching Wimbledon, investigating her family tree and generally enjoying being 'a lady that lunches', and fully enjoy the freedom after 42 years of full time work.

# Introduction

Gaining your qualification and becoming registered is just the start for any Dental Nurse or Dental Care Professional (DCP).

You have learnt all that theory and gained practical experience and you are now a qualified and registered DCP. Suddenly you are expected to know what to do in any situation. Where do you go for advice? What do you turn if you need answers immediately?

This *Survival Guide* series aims to be the resource that will help answer those questions. It is designed to be concise, with short brief answers to some questions and scenarios which will give immediate help.

I have tried to cover the most common situations but I am sure that I have missed some but hopefully these will be the exception rather than the rule. What is important is that you do not do anything outside your scope of practice and experience. The General Dental Council (GDC) has produced a *Scope of Practice* for DCP's which sets out what DCP's can, and cannot, do in professional practice. You should be fully conversant with these and should not undertake any duty or practice which falls outside this scope no matter who asks you to do so.

It is a fact that there is no substitute for experience and as you gain this experience, the problems and scenarios in this book will become routine, however there will be more to take their place.

Newly qualified nurses should not be embarrassed to ask their more experienced colleagues for help. Any experienced nurse will be only too happy to pass on their knowledge. Dentistry is about working as a team and the role of dental nurses are central to this. No dental practice or facility can work without a good team of dental nurses.

## References:

General Dental Council (2008) *Scope of Practice for Dental Care Professionals*

# SECTION I
# CLINICAL PRACTICE

# CHAPTER 1

# Dealing with medical emergencies

- **What should I do in a medical emergency?**
- **What drugs and equipment should the practice have available for medical emergencies?**
- **What should I do to avoid a medical emergency?**
- **What should I do when an emergency occurs?**
- **What are the common medical emergencies I might encounter?**
- **What are the more serious but infrequent emergencies I might encounter?**
- **What should I do in specific emergencies?**
- **Where can I get more information?**

## What should I do in a medical emergency?

It is important to recognise that serious medical emergencies are a rare occurrence in the dental surgery. However, this does not mean that the possibility should be ignored.

It is essential that all staff in the practice, not just the clinical staff, are aware of what to do if an emergency arises. It would be good practice to hold regular drills in the procedure to follow, which should include all the practice staff – dentists, dental nurses, reception staff, practice manager and hygienist if working onsite. It would be advisable for one person to be designated to take responsibility for ensuring that all emergency equipment, particularly drugs, are in date and in good condition. There must be emergency drugs available in every practice which are kept readily available in an emergency. There should also be at least one full oxygen cylinder; it would be better to have two so that there is a backup if one runs out. It would also be advisable to have a Automated External Defibrillator (AED) available. If the practice regularly carries out treatment under sedation, then a pulse oximeter, the machine routinely used to monitor a patients' pulse and oxygen saturation, should already be on site. Some more sophisticated monitors can also record electrocardiograms (ECG) for heart conditions.

## What drugs and equipment should the practice have available for medical emergencies?

Listed below are the essential types of drugs the practice should have available to deal with emergencies. Further information can be obtained from the *British National Formulary* (BNF).

**Glyceryl trinitrate** (GTN) **spray** – 400 micrograms per dose
This should be available for any patient who is being actively treated for angina. The patient should always carry their own but there are occasions when they forget and it should be available if the patient has an attack.

**Salbutamol inhaler** – 100 micrograms per actuation
This is a non specific inhaler that can be used by any asthmatic who has an attack requiring medication and does not have their own inhaler available. It can also be given to a patient who has respiratory distress but is not a diagnosed asthmatic or someone who is experiencing an anaphylactic attack.

**Adrenaline injection** – 1:1000 1 milligram per millilitre
For use by a trained practitioner for a patient who is having an anaphylactic shock.

**Aspirin dispersible** – 300 micrograms
Can be given to a patient suspected of having a myocardial infarction.

**Glucagon injection** – 1 milligram
Used in the treatment of unconscious hypoglycaemia.

**Oral glucose solution** – tablets, gel or powder
For a conscious diabetic having a hypoglycaemic attack.

**Midazolam** – 10 microgram per millilitre (buccal or intranasal)
To be administered by a trained professional to a patient having a prolonged epileptic attack.

Other equipment that should be available for medical emergencies include:

*Oxygen cylinders*: For administration to any patient having a medical emergency.

*Blood pressure machine*: To check blood pressure of a patient having a suspected cardiac incident.

*Automated External Defibrillator* (AED): To be used by trained personal to a patient who has suffered a cardiac arrest and the heart has stopped beating.

*Blood glucose monitor*: To check blood glucose levels of a patient suffering a hypoglycaemic attack and to monitor recovery after administering glucose.

*Pulse oximeter* (If sedation is carried out in the practice): To monitor heart rate and oxygen saturation and with more sophisticated models monitoring electro cardiac activity.

## What should I do to avoid a medical emergency?

It is essential that a detailed medical history is taken, checked at every visit and updated as necessary for every patient. This will give warning of known conditions and medication that should be taken, i.e. patients with known angina should always carry their own GTN spray which can be kept at hand during treatment; diabetic patients can be given a glucose drink if they haven't eaten for a while. Known allergies can also help to forestall anaphylactic incidents i.e. known latex allergy.

All dental professionals are required to complete 10 hours of verifiable Continued Professional Development (CPD) within each 5 year cycle on the subject of Medical Emergencies and Cardiopulmonary Resuscitation (CPR). It would be ideal to include all practice staff in this training and it is possible to have onsite training. Although this may cost more, it would provide a more pertinent training situation and could be used to refine the practice policies and procedures. If one member of staff is designated as having responsibility for emergency equipment then they should regularly check the Resuscitation Council's website (www.resus.org.uk) as the guidance they give is constantly being reviewed and revised.

## What should I do when an emergency occurs?

As soon as a patient says that they feel unwell or look unwell, then immediate action is required. Should an emergency occur it is essential that action is taken immediately and that a team approach is taken to ensure the best possible treatment for the patient. It should also be remembered that it isn't only the patient that may have a medical emergency, an escort may also be unwell, and so it is important that reception staff are alert to the procedures to be followed.

1. It is important to remember to:
- Stay calm.
- Ensure both your colleague's and your own safety.
- Put your medical emergency procedure into action.

2. If the patient is conscious:
- Ask – *'how are you?'*
- If they respond normally their airway will be clear and they will be breathing normally. Monitor them and check any relevant medical history. If they speak in short sentences they may have breathing problems.

3. If the patient is unresponsive:
- Shake them by the shoulders and ask *'are you all right'?*
- If the patient does not respond check breathing and pulse. If neither are present start cardiopulmonary resuscitation (CPR) according to latest recommendations.

In any medical emergency a systematic approach is essential. Use the ABCDE process to assess the patient.

### A (Airway)
– Check for airway obstruction.
– Head tilt, chin lift/jaw thrust.
– Remove visible debris.

- Use airway adjuncts e.g. oropharangeal airway.
- Give oxygen at 10 – 15 litres per minute.

## B (Breathing)
- Assess breathing.
- If not breathing, start basic life support.
- If breathing, count rate.
- Check chest expansion: is it equal on both sides?
- Is there a noise is it on inspiration or expiration?

## C (Circulation)
- Check pulse.
- If no pulse start CPR immediately.
- Check pulse rate.
- Check skin colour for pallor or flush.
- Check if the patient is warm or cold.
- Check blood pressure.
- Check capillary refill time.

## D (Disability)
- Assess level of consciousness.
- AVPU scale (Alert/Verbal/Painful/Unresponsive).
- Assess patient's central nervous system.
- Check pupil reaction using dental light.

## E (Exposure)
- Check for rashes or oedema.

This initial assessment should give sufficient information to provide appropriate treatment. It is also good practice to record the time and results of each assessment as well as the time delay from the first alert. This will be helpful to the paramedics if they are called.

## What are the common medical emergencies I might encounter?

Medical emergencies which occur more commonly in dental surgeries include:

### Asthma attacks
The stress of having dental treatment may cause an asthmatic to suffer an attack or they may react to chemical fumes in the surgery or practice.

### Hypoglycaemic attacks
Diabetic patients who are not well controlled may have a hypoglycaemic attack at any time, but the stress of having dental treatment may trigger an attack. Patients will sometimes not eat prior to an appointment in the mistaken belief that this is the right thing to do, which will lead to a dip in their blood glucose levels. Patients who have to wait for treatment may go past their usual eating time and have an attack.

### Syncope (fainting)
A lot of patients are frightened of having dental treatment. They do not eat prior to treatment and their blood sugar levels fall causing clammy feeling and sweating leading to faint.

### Angina
There are a large number of patients who are diagnosed with angina, who take medication and are normally fine. However going to the dentist is a stressful situation and this can cause extra pressure on the heart, by way of increased blood pressure which can trigger an angina attack

## What are the more serious but infrequent emergencies I might encounter?

### Anaphylaxis
This is an extreme response by the body to the introduction of a substance which the body is allergic to. Patients can be allergic to many substances and only have a minor rash or irritation if they come into contact with that substance. However some patients have an extreme reaction to a substance they are allergic to and actually collapse. The reaction causes swelling of the lungs and an inability to breathe. Such a reaction requires immediate attention and transfer to hospital. Dentists have to be particularly aware of patients who have a severe latex allergy, as they will need to wear non latex gloves and masks and use non latex rubber dam and local anaesthetic cartridges with non latex bungs.

## Epileptic seizures
Patients who are diagnosed epileptics can be well or poorly controlled. Well controlled patients will normally not present a problem but poorly controlled epileptics can have an attack triggered by the stress of attending a dentist.

## Adrenal insufficiency
Patients with adrenal insufficiency (sometimes known as Addison's Disease), lack a hormone, adrenaline, which is secreted into the blood stream in times of stress. As with other conditions, a well controlled patient will present no problems until you want to carry out an extraction or surgical procedure, when the body will require a larger amount. Dentists should consider advising patients to take an extra dose both pre and post op to accommodate this.

## Myocardial infarction
This is a heart attack in simple terms. Any patient with a known heart condition, angina or has previously had heart surgery or incidents should be carefully monitored during treatment and urged to advise the dentist or nurse if they feel at all unwell.

# What should I do in specific medical emergencies?

Specific medical emergencies may include:

## Asthma

1. Mild attack: The patient can use their own inhaler, repeated as necessary.
2. Severe attack: If the patient does not respond to their own medication, arrange for transfer to hospital by ambulance immediately.

### Signs and symptoms

1. Acute severe asthma attack in adults:
    - Inability to complete sentences in one breath.
    - Respiratory rate >25 per minute.

- Tachycardia (heart rate > 110 per minute).
2. Life threatening asthma attack in adults:
   - Cyanosis or a respiratory rate <8 per minute.
   - Bradycardia (heart rate < 50 per minute).
   - Exhaustion, confusion, decreased level of consciousness.

### Treatment

- CALL AN AMBULANCE IMMEDIATELY.
- Give oxygen at 10 – 15 litres per minute.
- 4 – 6 activations of salbutamol inhaler repeated every 10 minutes.
- If asthma is part of an anaphylactic reaction, give adrenaline injection.
- If patient becomes unresponsive, check breathing and circulation and start CPR.

## Anaphylaxis

A severe, life threatening, generalised or systematic hypersensitivity reaction. Patients who have a known severe allergic reaction may carry an EPIPEN for self administration. All patients who suffer an anaphylactic reaction must be sent to hospital for assessment, irrespective of level of recovery. Great care must be taken if treating children.

### Signs and symptoms

- Urticaria, erythema, rhinitis, conjunctivitis.
- Abdominal pain, vomiting, diarrhoea and a sense of impending doom.
- Flushing is common, but pallor may occur.
- Marked upper airway (laryngeal) oedema.
- Broncospasm causing stridor, wheezing and or hoarse voice.
- Vasodilation leading to low blood pressure and collapse. Possible cardiac arrest.
- Respiratory arrest leading to cardiac arrest.

*Dealing with medical emergencies*

### Treatment

- CALL AN AMBULANCE IMMEDIATELY.
- Use ABCDE assessment.
- Manage airway and breathing.
- Restore blood pressure.
- Lay patient flat and raise feet.
- Give oxygen at 10 – 15 litres per minute.
- In severe cases, give adrenaline 1:1000 injection intramuscularly.

## Angina

Cardiac (heart) condition. Known angina sufferers will carry their own GTN spray or tablets and should be allowed to use them initially.

### Signs and symptoms

- Chest pain.
- Shortness of breath.
- Fast or slow heart rate.
- Increased respiratory rate.
- Low blood pressure.
- Increased capillary refill time.
- Altered mental state.

### Treatment

- Administer GTN spray or tablet.
- If there is an immediate improvement then hospitalisation is not normally necessary.
- If there is no improvement after a second dose of spray or tablet, then an ambulance should be called and an ABCDE assessment should be carried out.

## Myocardial infarction

Cardiac (heart) attack.

### Signs and symptoms

- Pain similar to angina but more severe and prolonged.
- Unresponsive or partially responsive to GTN.
- Progressive severe crushing chest pain radiating to shoulders and down the arms, into the neck and jaw and through to the back.
- Pale, clammy skin.
- Nausea and vomiting.
- Weak pulse and low blood pressure.
- Shortness of breath.

### Treatment

- CALL AN AMBULANCE IMMEDIATELY.
- Allow the patient to rest in whatever position feels comfortable to them.
- Unconscious patients should be laid flat.
- Give high flow oxygen at 10 – 15 litres per minute.
- Give GTN spray if not already given.
- Reassure the patient if conscious.
- Give aspirin orally and let ambulance staff know that aspirin has been given.
- If the patient becomes unresponsive, check breathing and circulation and start CPR if necessary.

## Epileptic seizures

Known epileptics should take their medication as usual prior to dental treatment. Recognising epileptic seizures in patients who do not divulge their condition is easily achieved.

*Dealing with medical emergencies*

### Signs and symptoms

- May have a warning or 'aura'.
- Loss of consciousness, becomes giddy, falls and becomes cyanosed (tonic phase).
- This is followed by jerking limb movements and the tongue may be bitten (clonic phase).
- There may be frothing of the mouth and urinary incontinence.
- This typically lasts a few minutes, then the patient may become floppy but remain unconscious.
- Patient will regain consciousness after a varying time but may be confused.
- Fitting may also be a sign of hypoglycaemia and should be considered in known diabetics. If possible a blood glucose measurement should be taken.
- Check for a slow heart rate (< 40 per minute) which causes low blood pressure, and may cause a transient cerebral hypoxia and give rise to a brief fit. This can be the result of a vasovagal attack also.

### Treatment

- Reassure the patient and move any equipment away from patient to remove risk of injury.
- Do not attempt to put anything in the patient's mouth or between the teeth.
- Do not attempt to use any airway adjuncts.
- Give oxygen at 10 – 15 litres per minute.
- Do not restrain convulsive movements.
- When convulsions cease, put patient in the recovery position and reassess.
- If patient remains unresponsive, check breathing and circulation and start CPR.
- Check blood glucose level to eliminate hypoglycaemia. If suspected give glucose orally or buccally.
- After convulsion ceases, reassure the patient and do not discharge until fully recovered and accompanied home.
- Transfer to hospital is not always necessary unless seizures are atypical (unusual) or prolonged or an injury is sustained. If seizures

are prolonged or recur in rapid succession, call an ambulance.
- Ambulance staff will give medication but a less effective treatment is the administration of buccal or intranasal midazolam (10 mg for adults). The dental nurse should not routinely administer this however if alone and confident in what they are doing, they could administer a dose whilst waiting for assistance.

### Hypoglycaemia

Known diabetics should eat, drink and take their normal medication prior to dental treatment. If the blood glucose level falls to <3.0 mmol per litre, then they become hypoglycaemic, although this can happen at higher levels in some patients. Patients will often recognise the symptoms themselves and will respond quickly to glucose.

#### Signs and symptoms

- Shaking and trembling.
- Sweating.
- Headache.
- Difficulty in concentrating and vagueness.
- Slurring of speech.
- Aggression or confusion.
- Fitting.
- Unconsciousness.

#### Treatment

- Confirm diagnosis by measuring blood glucose levels.

1. Early Stages
- Patient is co-operative, conscious and there is an intact gag reflex.
- Give oral glucose and repeat every 10 – 15 minutes if necessary.

2. Severe Cases
- Patient is unco-operative and unable to swallow safely.
- Give buccal glucose gel or glucagon.

*Dealing with medical emergencies*

- Glucagon is given intramuscularly and may take 5 – 10 minutes to work.
- It may be ineffective in anorexic patients, alcoholics and some non-diabetic patients.
- Recheck blood glucose level after 10 minutes.
- If patient becomes unconscious check breathing and circulation and begin CPR.

Once the patient becomes alert and able to swallow they should be given a drink containing glucose and some high carbohydrate food. Patient can go home if fully recovered and accompanied, but they should not drive.

## Syncope

Causes are attributed to inadequate cerebral perfusion and inadequate oxygenation. This results in loss of consciousness. It occurs with low blood pressure and is known as a vasovagal attack, syncope or simple faint.
Possible causes include:
- Postural hypotension – sitting patient up quickly or standing for too long. When sitting patients up after prolonged treatment in the supine position, do so in stages.
- Hyperventilation – rapid, shallow breathing by anxious patients may cause light headedness or faintness but does not usually result in syncope. Usually reassurance is all that is necessary.

### Signs and symptoms

- Feel faint, dizzy or light headed.
- Slow pulse rate.
- Low blood pressure.
- Pallor and sweating.
- Nausea and vomiting.
- Loss of consciousness.

### Treatment

- Immediately lie patient flat and elevate the legs.

- Loosen tight clothing and give oxygen at 10 – 15 litres per minute.
- If patient becomes unresponsive, check breathing and circulation and start CPR.

## Choking and aspiration

Patients are susceptible to choking during treatment but good teamwork and careful attention will reduce the risk.

### Signs and symptoms

- Patient may cough or splutter.
- Complain of difficulty in breathing.
- Noisy breathing:
  - Wheeze – Aspiration.
  - Stridor – Upper respiratory obstruction.
- May develop paradoxical chest or abdominal movements.
- Become cyanosed and lose consciousness.

### Treatment

- Aspiration – allow patient to cough vigorously.
- Treating a wheeze with salbutamol inhaler may help.
- Large pieces of foreign material (teeth or amalgam) - refer to hospital for chest X Ray and removal.
- If symptomatic after aspiration then refer to hospital.
- Choking patients should have the visible foreign body removed from the mouth and pharynx.
- Encourage coughing if conscious. If unable to cough but conscious, sharp back blows should be given, followed by abdominal thrusts if not dislodged.
- If patient becomes unconscious begin CPR. The pressure generated may dislodge the foreign body. Only circulatory support should be given unless the foreign body is dislodged.

### Adrenal insufficiency

This is a rare occurrence in the dental surgery and other causes must be considered in cases of collapse. This may follow long term administration of oral corticosteroids. The patient can become hypotensive in times of physiological stress.

#### Signs and symptoms

- Normal dental treatment should not pose a problem but surgical extractions or implant placements may pose problems as well as dental related infections.

#### Treatment

- It can be prevented by the patient taking an increased dose prior to treatment.
- In cases of collapse an increased prophylactic dose may be indicated.

Guidance for the treatment of such patients may be found on the Addison's Society website (www.addisons.org.uk).

## Where can I get more information?

The Resuscitation Council (2006) publish a booklet specifically written for dental professionals which gives indepth information on emergencies, training, drugs and equipment. They also publish flow charts within their guidance which can be printed and kept for quick reference. It is advisable that all dental practices should have a copy for reference but there is no substitute for training.

Another useful book to have in the practice and written specifically for dental care professionals is *The Management of Medical Emergencies: A guide for dental care professionals* (Balmer and Longman 2008).

This chapter cannot give exhaustive information and is only meant as a quick reference. There is no substitute for adequate, appropriate and regular training in medical emergencies and CPR.

## References

Addison's Society www.addisons.org.uk (accessed 28.1.2011)

Balmer, C and Longman, L (2008) *The Management of Medical Emergencies: A guide for dental care professionals*, Quay Books, London

British National Formulary website http://bnf.org/bnf/index.htm (accessed 28.1.2011)

Resuscitation Council (2006) *Standards for Clinical Practice and Training for Dental Practitioners and Dental Care Professionals in General Dental Practice*

Resuscitation Council www.resus.org.uk (accessed 28.1.2011)

# CHAPTER 2

# Dealing with dental emergencies

- **What are the common dental emergencies I might encounter?**
- **What should I do in specific dental emergencies?**
- **How can I ensure the surgery is ready for the emergency patient?**

## What are the common dental emergencies I might encounter?

Patients may present with a dental emergency and it is important that the correct actions are taken as soon as possible. The true dental emergencies are listed below:

1. Haemorrhage.
2. Facial trauma.
3. Avulsed teeth.
4. Swelling, intra-oral or extra-oral.

Dental pain is not a true dental emergency although a patient will believe it is and will need careful handling when this is pointed out to them. Even though dental pain is not a true emergency, provision will have to be made to treat these patients urgently.

## What should I do in specific dental emergencies?

### *Haemorrhage*

Dental haemorrhage is usually a result of a dental extraction or other surgical dental procedure.

### Treatment

- When a patient presents with a haemorrhage, they must be seen immediately.
- Take the patient into the surgery or a place where they can spit out and be away from other waiting patients.
- Reassure patient.
- Patient should not be left alone.
- The patient treatment record should be checked for relevant medical history and medication.
- Check the mouth and if appropriate, place a bite pack in the area and ask the patient to bite hard on it.
- Alert the dentist to the emergency and ensure they examine the patient as a matter of priority.
- Prepare suture equipment.
- If there is a relevant medical history, i.e. warfarin therapy or bleeding disorder, consider calling an ambulance.
- Assist whilst dentist treats haemorrhage.
- If haemorrhage continues refer to hospital.

## Facial trauma

This can be the result of a fall, a physical fight, motor accident etc. It is important to carefully examine the patient both extra and intra-orally. Radiographs will have to be taken to fully assess the extent of the trauma and to locate any pieces of broken teeth. Pieces of tooth may be in the lips or cheeks but all must be accounted for to rule out the possibility of them being inhaled.

### Treatment

- Emergency treatment must be carried out to any broken teeth; extraction of retained roots, removal of broken pieces that are still attached, extirpation of exposed pulp canals, smoothing of sharp edges etc.
- Suture any intra-oral soft tissue injuries.
- Diagnosis from radiographic evidence.
- Reassurance and explanation to the patient.

*Dealing with dental emergencies*

- Referrals to hospital for expert treatment if fractures are diagnosed or if there are extra oral facial injuries.

### Avulsed (knocked out) teeth

If a patient presents with a tooth that has been completely knocked out and is undamaged and they have the tooth, time is of the essence. There is a good chance of success if the tooth can be replaced within an hour of being knocked out.

### Treatment

- The tooth should not be scrubbed clean as this will remove remnants of tissue which are still attached. These remnants will help with successful reimplantation.
- The tooth may need to be splinted to give it support and protection during the healing process.
- The tooth will also need to be subject to regular checks to forestall problems.
- It may be necessary to carry out endodontic treatment on the tooth in the future.
- If a patient telephones for advice then the patient should be advised to:
    o Gently wash the tooth in clean water but do not scrub it.
    o If possible replace the tooth in its socket.
    o If not possible to replace, place in a container and cover it with milk.
    o Immediately present at the surgery.
- If a patient telephones for advice with a tooth knocked out of alignment but not completely out of the mouth, then the tooth should be gently pushed back into line and immediately present at the surgery for treatment.

### Swelling, intra-oral or extra-oral

Extra-oral facial swelling may not have a dental cause but if it is around the jaw or nose, then there are many potential causes which are listed below along with the initial treatment. In all cases immediate examination is essential with the use of radiographs to make an informed diagnosis. If in any doubt, urgent referral for specialist advice should be made.

### Treatment

- Fractured jaw – immediate referral to hospital.
- Post extraction swelling – analgesia and possibly antibiotics.
- Apical abscess – pulp extirpation and antibiotics or extraction.
- Periodontal abscess – irrigation of periodontal ligament antibiotics.
- Oral cancers – immediate urgent referral for specialist diagnosis and treatment.

Any soft tissue swelling of the tongue or cheeks without obvious relationship to a tooth must be investigated urgently. If there is evidence of white patches, the patient must be referred to a specialist as soon as can be arranged as this could be a sign of a possible tumour. It is essential that the patient is kept informed but not alarmed until a diagnosis is agreed.

## How can I ensure the surgery is ready for the emergency patient?

When you prepare the surgery/treatment room for the day, an efficient dental nurse will be prepared for the unexpected. Most practices will have appointments set aside for emergencies or patients who have problems. There are few true dental emergencies (see the ones outlined earlier).

However any patient that is in pain from losing a filling, crown, has a broken denture or sore gums will believe they have a dental emergency and want that problem treated immediately. Such patients may have to be fitted in between patients who are booked for routine treatment. The nurse must be prepared for such eventualities. This will require you to:

- Ensure instruments are decontaminated and sterilised as soon as they are finished with to ensure a constant supply.
- Be prepared for impressions to be taken.
- Be prepared to have equipment for opening and dressing a tooth.

*Dealing with dental emergencies*

- Be prepared for emergency extirpations.
- Have equipment ready for extractions.
- Be prepared to explain procedures to patients who will be upset and in pain and calm and defuse possible difficult situations.

Always remember that if a patient has a problem, it is an emergency to them, even if it isn't a true dental emergency. It is important to always be aware of their concerns and feelings.

# CHAPTER 3

# Dealing with daily practices

- **Can I work unsupervised when I am training?**
- **What am I allowed to do and not to do?**
- **What responsibilities will I have as a newly qualified dental nurse?**
- **What help should I expect to receive as a trainee?**
- **What procedures do I need to carry out to prepare the surgery at the start of the day?**
- **What decontamination procedures do I need to carry out between patients?**
- **What decontamination procedures do I need to carry out at the end of the patient sessions?**
- **What decontamination procedures do I need to carry out at the end of the day?**

Dental nursing is essentially a practical profession. You learn a lot of theory covering how the body works and things which will influence and affect how a dentist carries out dental treatment but as your career progresses a lot of this theoretical knowledge will be pushed to the back of your mind, replaced by practical knowledge gained from experience. It is this knowledge gained from experience that is needed by the trainee or newly qualified nurse and it is the experienced nurses around you in the workplace that can pass on theirs to you.

## Can I work unsupervised when I am training?

Since the advent of compulsory registration in 2008, it is illegal to employ an unqualified dental nurse unless they are registered on an accredited training scheme. Whilst undertaking this training it is advisable for a qualified nurse to be close by for advice and guidance. Experienced dental nurses can supplement the training of these nurses by giving them the benefit of their experience which is an invaluable addition to the textbook learning.

As a trainee dental nurse you should never be left without the backup of a qualified colleague. You should never be expected to assist with the treatment of patients under conscious sedation although you can gain valuable knowledge by acting as a runner for the qualified nurse. You should never be left to assist with the treatment of medically compromised patients. An ideal situation would be for you to have a designated qualified nurse to act as your mentor within the practice, someone you can turn to for advice and reassurance and someone who will explain why procedures were followed in emergency situations. This practice 'mentor' would be in addition to the tutor on the course that you are registered with.

## What am I allowed to do and not to do?

It is a complete culture shock when you get those two certificates that prove that you are qualified and are registered with the General Dental Council (GDC). All of a sudden you are expected to know everything and be able to deal with any situation. You are expected to take responsibility for your actions without having someone to supervise you. How do you know what you are supposed to do and what you are supposed not to do? Where do you turn for guidance?

A well run practice would work out a transitional plan so that you are inducted into everything expected of you in your new role as a qualified dental nurse. When this is arranged it would usually mean that the practice will continue to teach you and the other qualified nurses will support you. This is not always the case and you may well find that you expected to have the same responsibility as the more experienced nurses.

When you registered as a Dental Care Professional (DCP) with the GDC you will have received a copy of the GDC *Standards of Dental Professionals* (2008) which is essential reading for all DCP's and must be followed. Failure to do so could result in action being taken by the GDC which could result in your removal from the DCP register held by the GDC. This would mean that you could not be legally employed as a dental nurse.

*Daily working practices*

## What responsibilities will I have as a newly qualified dental nurse?

The list of duties that all dental professionals, including dental nurses, are allowed to carry out is contained within the GDC *Scope of Practice for Dental Nurses* (2008) document. In this document the role of a dental nurse is described as:-

*'Dental Nurses are registered Dental professionals who provide clinical and other support to other registrants and patients.'*

It goes on to list the basic duties and additional skills dental nurses could develop during their careers and additional skills on prescription. However it also states that:-

*'Dental Nurses do not diagnose disease or treatment plan. All other skills are reserved to one or more of the other registrant groups.'*

Dental nurses should restrict their work activities to those listed in the *Scope of Practice for Dental Nurses*. If you are asked to perform any task or take on any responsibility not on the list, you must refuse, to protect your registration.

The moment you get those certificates of qualification and registration, you go from trainee to qualified nurse. So what should you expect to be different?

- You will be expected to take responsibility for your own actions. It will no longer be acceptable to pass the problem to another team member.
- You must be sure that what you are saying or doing is right. If you are not sure, you must ask for help and admit that you are not sure.
- You can reasonably expect to have an induction into your new role and responsibility.
- It would be reasonable to expect one of the experienced nurses to act as your mentor to ensure you are not put into a position where your inexperience can put you or your patient in danger.

- You are a member of a professional team and you are as important as every other team member and you are entitled to play a full part in that team. This means that not only must every other team member involve you in what is going on, but you must also make sure you involve yourself.

Dental nurses must ensure their patients are cared for before, during and after treatment. You must concentrate on the needs of the patient as well as those of the dentist, so that the dentist can concentrate on achieving a high standard of dentistry.

Your role in assisting the dentist is pivotal to your job. It has been said that the working relationship between a dentist and dental nurse is as close as or even closer than that of a married couple. It is certain that there must be mutual respect to ensure an effective and efficient team. It is also certain that an efficient, qualified and registered dental nurse can make the difference between a practice keeping a full list of satisfied patients and failing completely.

Dentists should encourage their nurses to carry out their CPD effectively and should involve them in training on new practices, equipment and materials which they intend to use when working chair side. When working chairside, you must always be alert to the needs of the patient and the dentist. In general you will be required to:

- Keep the work field clear.
- Retract soft tissues with the aspirator.
- Aspirate water / saliva from the mouth.
- Ensure the patient is protected from excess water escaping from the mouth.
- Watch for signs of discomfort – screwing up eyes, wincing etc.
- Comfort the patient whilst a local anaesthetic is given.
- Reassure the patient and ensure they understand what is happening.
- Clear treatment area effectively.
- Be alert to the needs of the dentist:
    o Pass instruments
    o Have materials ready for use
    o Keep the work area clear and tidy.
- Prepare for the next patient.
- Decontaminate and sterilise the instruments.
- Ensure there is no chance of cross contamination between patients.

*Daily working practices*

## What help should I expect to receive as a trainee?

As a trainee registered on an accredited course, you will receive tutor support as you work towards your qualification. As well as lectures, they will monitor your progress in your practical work which is completed within your workplace. In a general practice this will be given by all the other qualified members of staff. If you work in a larger institution, such as a dental hospital, you will receive closer support because the tutors will be on site all the time. In a practice you will most probably only visit the college on one day a week when you can receive help from your tutor.

The qualified nurses in the practice must be prepared to pass on their expertise based on their hands-on experience and knowledge. You must not be afraid to ask for assistance with new techniques, materials and procedures. You should also ask them to explain the reasons they do things in a particular way so that you can learn.

The onus is very much on you to ask for this help. The qualified nurses will know that a trainee nurse will need help but they will assume that a newly qualified nurse will only need minimal advice. You cannot expect your colleagues to know when you need help, you must be prepared to ask questions or query why they do something in the way that they do.

The experienced nurse must be prepared to explain why you are working in the way you do or have the standards you have to follow. The presence of a newly qualified or trainee nurse in your practice or clinic makes the need for regular team meetings even more paramount.

## What procedures do I need to carry out to prepare the surgery at the start of the day?

In 2008 a document entitled *Health Technical Memorandum 01-05, Decontamination in Primary Dental Care* (HTM 01-05) was published by the Department of Health which gives detailed guidelines for decontamination standards which are enforceable by law.

The whole surgery area must be considered to be either contaminated or at risk of contamination, therefore the whole area must be decontaminated at the start of the day. You will be required to:

29

- Ensure that all devices are switched on at the mains (compressor, suction apparatus, dental chair and unit, accessory equipment) as appropriate.
- Put on protective clothing to cover your uniform (plastic apron, heavy duty rubber gloves and protective eye wear).
- To comply with HTM 01-05, all mains fed water lines must be flushed for a minimum of 2 minutes. Any waterlines fed from bottled water supply should be flushed for 30 secs or to the manufacturer's instructions. This must be done prior to wiping down as an aerosol is produced which may be contaminated and a mask should be worn to avoid inhalation of the aerosol. It is essential that all and every waterline in the chair and unit is flushed at the start of every session.
- Make up fresh detergent or disinfectant solutions to manufacturer's instructions.
- Wipe down all surfaces of the dental chair and unit as well as work surfaces and cupboard fronts, with a detergent or disinfectant solution as recommended by the manufacturer's instructions for the equipment. Any disinfectant solution used must be capable of killing bacteria, viruses, and fungi.
- When all wiping down has been completed, remove protective clothing and dispose of disposable items in the clinical waste.
- Put on clean examination gloves and complete preparation of the surgery and treatment area.
- A system of 'zoning' should be employed to reduce the amount of decontamination required between patients. This entails having contaminated zones and clean zones. Contaminated zones should only have contaminated items placed in them and clean zones reserved for non-contaminated items.
- Contaminated zones should be covered with inpermeable, disposable covers i.e. light handles, tubings, triple syringe handles, chair controls (if not foot operated) etc.
- Clean areas can be covered by a disposable paper sheet.
- When everything has been wiped down and covered, then put out the equipment needed for the first patient. Do not put out equipment that cannot be sterilised in the aerosol zone. This is the zone approximately 2 metres from the patient's head, in all directions.
- Put out medicaments and materials required in the clean area.
- Patient paper treatment notes or the computer must also be kept out

*Daily working practices*

of the aerosol zone and the computer keyboard should, ideally, be wipable and easily decontaminated. Care should be taken when using computer keyboards or writing up notes that contaminated gloves are removed and hand hygiene carried out.
- Once the surgery area has been prepared then the decontamination/ sterilisation area must be prepared. The ultrasonic bath should be filled with the appropriate solution, the washer disinfector should be tested and prepared for use and the autoclave prepared and tested prior to use.
- Check that all and every item that may be required for the session are available. A robust ordering and stock control system is essential for the efficient working of the practice.

## What decontamination procedures do I need to carry out between patients?

Once the treatment has been completed and the patient has left the treatment area, it must be fully decontaminated prior to the next patient entering. This is when efficient 'zoning' will prove invaluable to you. If you have successfully 'zoned' then the only areas that will need thorough decontamination are those that have been contaminated during treatment. If 'zoning' has not been efficient, then all areas will require very careful and thorough decontamination. As you become more experienced, you will learn to clear your work areas as you go along and keep the work areas as uncluttered as possible.

To decontaminate an area, follow these steps:

- Using heavy duty rubber gloves, remove all contaminated instruments, handpieces, accessory items and disposable covers.
- Put the equipment into the designated decontamination sink, in the decontamination area, taking care to remove them in a safe manner.
- Put all used disposable items into the clinical waste bags, except 'sharps' which must be disposed of in the appropriate sharps container.
- Flush through all water lines for 30 seconds and aspirate clean water through the suction apparatus.
- Wipe down all contaminated surfaces with a recommended

disinfectant that has bactericidal, virucidal and fungicidal properties.
- Disinfect any unsterilisable items i.e. protective glasses.
- Remove gloves, perform hand hygiene and put on clean examination gloves and put out fresh covers, disposable items and equipment needed for the next patient.
- The contaminated items that were used have to be thoroughly decontaminated using either an ultrasonic bath or a washer/disinfector prior to sterilisation in an autoclave. Ideally this will be done by a second person while you work chairside with the next patient. If there is no second person available, then you will need to evolve a system of working both at chairside and in the decontamination area.
- It is essential that no contaminated item is used on another patient if it has not been sterilised.

## What decontamination procedures do I need to carry out at the end of the patient session?

At the end of the session the surgery should be cleaned as described above. Additionally:

- All 'clean zones' must be thoroughly wiped over with detergent solution followed by an appropriate disinfectant. Protective clothing should be worn.
- Good ventilation of the area is essential at this time to dissipate any harmful fumes.
- Disinfect any items that are to be sent to a laboratory and complete the necessary paperwork prior to collection or posting to the laboratory.
- Any items for repair should be decontaminated if possible and prepared for collection or posting with the appropriate paperwork.
- The area can be prepared for the start of the next session if this is only a brief break, i.e. lunch.
- If the end of this session is the end of the day then further decontamination is required.

*Daily working practices*

## What decontamination procedures do I need to carry out at the end of the day?

- Follow the procedure for the 'end of session' as outlined previously.
- All accessory equipment should be decontaminated thoroughly as per the manufacturer's instructions and put away.
- All electrical accessory equipment should be unplugged, decontaminated and stored away.
- The computer should be closed down and turned off at the mains and then wiped down with appropriate decontaminants.
- All work surfaces and equipment must be cleaned with detergent followed by a suitable disinfectant.
- If bottled water is used, then the manufacturer's instructions must be followed. Some will call for bottles to be emptied and left empty overnight, others say that the bottles can be left filled. Whatever the instructions are, they must be followed carefully.
- Some instructions will call for the use of a bleach solution, sodium hypochlorite at a concentration of 1000 parts per million, or 10,000 parts per million for blood spillages. If this is used then it should be left to lie on surfaces for about 30 minutes or for as long as possible.
- Aspirators must be run through with a suitable surfactant as recommended by the manufacturers. These solutions help to break down biofilms which can build up in tubings, as well as remove fresh bacteria. Solutions used should be non-foaming, household detergents will not suffice. If a foaming solution is used, it will damage the internal workings of the equipment.
- Newer dental units may have a built in system for decontaminating the internal workings of the handpiece tubings, aspirator and spittoon. If these are available in your dental unit, then they should be used to ensure efficient disinfection of all the unit.
- If the aspiration system you have is a portable system, it is impossible to effectively clean and disinfect the mechanism of the unit. The disposal of the contents of the bottle pose a considerable risk and advice should be sort as to local regulations to putting the contents into the sewerage system. For these reasons the use of portable aspiration systems is not advised.
- All clinical waste must be prepared for collection as per the local regulations.

*Dental Nurse Survival Guide*

- All equipment, instruments, handpieces etc that have been used and can be sterilised, must be decontaminated thoroughly and sterilised prior to leaving at the end of the day. They should be either packed after sterilisation or stored in clean receptacles overnight. No contaminated items should be left in a contaminated state overnight.
- Once the surgery has been completely decontaminated and closed down, then the decontamination area must also be cleaned down and closed down.
- Ultrasonic baths must be emptied, wiped out and unplugged from the mains.
- Washer/disinfectors must be closed down in accordance with manufacturer's instructions.
- Autoclave reservoirs must be emptied and dried out and the door of the chamber left open, dry and clean. They should be turned off and unplugged.
- All work surfaces should be cleaned down with a recommended disinfectant, as should any other equipment in the area i.e. oil cans etc.
- Before leaving the building, check that all equipment is switched off as required and that everything is left in a safe state.

During any decontamination/sterilisation procedures, appropriate protective equipment must be worn at all times and disposed of appropriately. You should be aware of changing from heavy duty to examination gloves and the need for hand hygiene to be carried out. The very last thing that should be done when leaving the surgery is to effectively wash your hands.

For more detailed information on all aspects of infection prevention, control and decontamination techniques, there is a book specifically designed and written for dental nurses covering all these issues (Porter 2008). Copies of HTM 01-05 have been distributed to all dental facilities, along with a self assessment tool to check your compliance You should ensure that you have a working knowledge of the contents of the document. The dentist in charge of your practice will have ultimate responsibility for ensuring that the standards and recommendations are complied with but the day to day responsibility for carrying out the tasks will fall in a large part, to you. You should ensure that you fully understand what is outlined and that you work to them. You should not be persuaded to cut corners and should ensure that you do not let your standards slip.

# References

General Dental Council (2008) *Standards for Dental Professionals*

General Dental Council (2008) *Scope of Practice for Dental Nurses*

Department of Health - Dental Practices (2008) *Health Technical Memorandum 01-05 – Decontamination in Primary Dental Care*

Porter, K (2008) *A Dental Nurses Guide to Infection Control and Decontamination* Quay Books, London

# CHAPTER 4

# Preventing cross infection

- **What are the basic principles of preventing cross infection?**
- **What legal obligations do I have?**
- **What are the common infections I need to protect against?**
- **What should I do to protect myself?**
- **What Personal Protective Equipment (PPE) should I use?**
- **How do I ensure I effectively wash my hands?**
- **When should I wash my hands?**
- **How else can I ensure I carry out effective hand hygiene?**
- **Is my personal hygiene important?**
- **What should I do if I have a 'sharps' injury?**
- **Who else can I rely on to protect me?**

## What are the basic principles of preventing cross infection?

The basic standards on infection control for healthcare workers, known as *Standard Precautions*, were first introduced as *Universal Precautions* in 1987 by the Centre for Disease Control and Prevention (CDC) based in Atlanta USA. They were initially issued as recommendations for the prevention of the spread of the Human Immunodeficiency Virus (HIV). This document outlined precautions to be taken to protect both patients and health care workers for the first time from the spread of infection. It emphasised that these precautions must be consistently used **for all patients** irrespective of known infectivity. It outlined the precautions that should be taken:

- Use of Personal Protective Equipment (PPE), including gloves, masks, goggles or face shields, gowns or disposable aprons.
- Effective and timely hand washing.

- Prevention of needlestick injuries.
- Use of shields if giving mouth to mouth resuscitation.
- Routine covering of all skin wounds.

The document outlined extra precautions to be taken in dentistry and stated that:

*"Blood, saliva and gingival fluid from ALL patients should be considered infective'. CDC 1987*

It went on to advocate the use of rubber dam, high speed aspiration and outlined the correct positioning of the patient to reduce the generation of aerosols. It described the need for the sterilisation of handpieces, the need for the flushing of waterlines and the thorough and careful disinfection of all items to be sent to a laboratory. It was the first document to advocate the covering of surfaces that cannot be sterilised.

The *Universal Precautions* were updated in 1996 and renamed *Standard Precautions*. It was felt that 'universal' implied perfection and although comprehensive these precautions could not provide perfect protection.

In 2003 the British Dental Association (BDA) updated the *Standard Precautions* and made them more relevant to current dental practice to include:

- The use of PPE.
- Effective hand washing.
- Safe disposal of sharps.
- Safe disposal of clinical waste.
- Effective hard surface decontamination.
- Effective decontamination and sterilisation of contaminated items.
- Use of zoning techniques to prevent contamination of unsterilisable items.
- Safe storage of sterilised items.

*Standard Precautions* should also be followed by any person that comes into contact with contaminated items. It should also be remembered that some infectious diseases are more infectious before they show external symptoms therefore *Standard Precautions* must be followed for every patient that attends for treatment.

*Preventing cross infection*

As well as implementing cleaning and decontaminating processes there has been a growing number of disposable items used in dental practice to ensure against contamination. The use of disposable items are an essential part of *Standard Precautions* as long as they are disposed of correctly, i.e. in clinical waste. This is being extended into the manufacture of disposable instruments. Disposable items must only be used once and carry a symbol to designate this fact (see *Figure 4.1*):

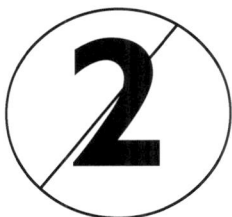

Figure 4.1 Symbol denoting single use item.

You should never use an item marked with this symbol on a second occasion and they should not be sterilised. There are some products marked with this symbol which can be sterilised prior to use and thrown away after use. Such items are fine bore aspirator tips that may be used in a surgical procedure and are not supplied in a sterile state. However sterile narrow bore aspirators are available and should be the product of choice.

The Medicines and Healthcare Products Regulatory Agency (MHRA) regularly publishes guidance and updates on the use of medical devices (instruments etc). The dentist should receive notification of these alerts. They are published if there are a large number of failures of a particular medical device where users need to be aware of potential problems. The dental nurse needs to be informed if the alert gives advice as to the decontamination of a device or other restrictions in its use. The dentist is also duty bound to report to the MHRA any failure of a medical device, i.e. if an instrument breaks it must be retained and the breakage reported to the MHRA, so that the MHRA can investigate if there are a large number of breakages of that particular item.

The BDA also published the *Infection Control in Dentistry Advice Sheet A12* in 2003 which gave dental practices detailed advice on how to follow these *Standard Precautions*. This outlined specific precautions which had to be followed for patients with known infections such as:

- Prior contaminations (Creutzfeldt-Jakob Disease (CJD) and variant Creutzfeldt-Jakob Disease (vCJD))
- Airborne transmissable diseases (tuberculosis)
- Droplet transmissable diseases (mumps, influenza)
- Transmission by direct or indirect contact with dried skin (Colonisation by MRSA or contaminated surfaces)

This advice booklet was superceded by the *Health Technical Memorandum 01-05* (HTM 01-05) which was introduced by the Department of Health in 2008. The HTM 01-05 is now the document of choice to consult on all areas concerned with infection prevention and control and decontamination. A self assessment tool was also supplied with the hard copies of the document when it was supplied to each and every dental institution in 2008. This self assessment tool was devised by The Infection Prevention Society (IPS) and is updated regularly. It provides an invaluable tool in assessing how compliant your practice is with the new regulations. It is the tool used by auditors who visit to carry out the audit required by the HTM 01-05.

The HTM 01-05 also sets out Essential Quality Requirements (EQR) which are the standards that should be complied with now and Best Practice (BP) which are the standards which must be achieved in the future. Failure to meet the standards set out in EQR could mean that a practice is closed until improvements are made. Written plans on how the practice will achieve BP must be in place when the practice is audited.

## What legal obligations do I have?

Even though you are not responsible, legally, for what happens in the practice, you should be aware of the laws that have been enacted to protect your patients, your colleagues and yourself from Healthcare Acquired Infections (HCAI).

The primary legislation setting out basic rules for all healthcare establishments is The Health Act 2006 (DoH). It relates to the provision of healthcare directly by NHS organisations and is presented under three headings:

1. NHS organisations have a general duty of care ensuring that appropriate

management systems are in place to protect patients, staff and others from Healthcare Acquired Infections (HCAI).
2. Relates to clinical procedures placing a duty of care on NHS organisations to adhere to care policies applicable to the prevention and control of HCAI.
3. NHS organisations have a duty to ensure as far as possible that healthcare workers are free of, and protected from, exposure to communicable infections during the course of their work. They must also have the necessary education to prevent and control HCAI.

Working in a dental practice, you are also bound by certain other laws and regulations, all of which are regularly reviewed and revised. It is imperative that you, or someone in your practice, keeps an eye on these changes because any breaches of their regulations could have severe consequences as these are enforceable by law. The following is a brief summary of the more important pieces of legislation:

1. *The Health and Safety at Work Act 1974*
   This Act sets out a framework that places a duty of care upon employers and employees to promote high standards in the workplace as well as protecting the public from workplace dangers.

2. *Management of Health and Safety at Work Regulations 1999*
   These regulations take into law the requirements of the European Union directives which address issues of training, risk assessment and development of health and safety policies. Further additions to the regulations required employers to put in place preventative and protective measures and made it possible for an employer to be prosecuted for the actions of an employee.

3. *Control of Substances Hazardous to Health 1988* (COSHH)
   These are regulations designed to prevent substances used in the workplace from causing harm to people working with them or patients being treated using them. It requires that all and any substances have a risk assessment carried out before they are used and that these assessments are written recorded and revised regularly. The assessment should include maximum safe exposure limits and any first aid and follow up treatments that are required if exposure occurs.

4. *Environmental Protection Act* (1990)
   This Act sets out the legal guidelines for the safe disposal of waste in all forms, especially contaminated waste and clinical waste. It also sets out rules for the safe disposal of substances such as mercury and amalgam.

Many of the requirements set out in these acts of legislation are brought together with other guidelines and standards in the HTM 01-05.

## What are the common infections I need to protect against?

It is imperative that you protect yourself against the many infections that are carried by patients, other staff, visitors or escorts. All dental nurses must be vaccinated against blood borne viruses, the main one being hepatitis B. This is currently the only hepatitis variant that can be vaccinated against. The other major consideration is HIV/AIDS but there is, as yet, no vaccination available against this.

These are the most notorious infections that are of concern to dental professionals and it is essential that all dental nurses are vaccinated against hepatitis B and that your immunity level is regularly checked and boosted if necessary.

Other infections which are beginning to become more prevalent are measles, mumps, rubella and tuberculosis. These are infections that can be avoided by vaccination but the uptake of vaccination for children has fallen off significantly following adverse publicity about possible side effects.

Many of these infections are at their most contagious before the visible signs or symptoms are apparent. Reasonable precautions to protect yourself against this possible threat are essential and advice about boosters and immunity levels sought from either your General Medical Practitioner (GMP) or your local Occupational Health Department (OHD). You are responsible primarily for protecting yourself. This may come at a monetary cost as some GPs will charge for these injections. The practice you work for may be willing to help out with these expenses or may have an arrangement with a local GP but if they don't you will have to cover the cost yourself. This should not be an excuse for not maintaining your protection levels.

## What should I do to protect myself?

You must have your immunity levels checked regularly and booster injections arranged should your immunity be in doubt. This will involve having a blood test which should be arranged through your local OHD who will give advice on the best course of action after the results are known.

It is possible for some people to not gain immunity after a course of hepatitis B injections. This does not preclude you from working at the chairside but you must take extra care and be scrupulous in your adherence to *Standard Precautions*.

It is almost impossible to protect yourself completely against infections that may be brought in by patients or their escorts. Patients will not know if they are incubating infections, they may not feel ill or show any visible signs such as spots or rashes. It becomes imperative that *Standard Precautions* are scrupulously adhered to for every patient that attends. It is also important that other public areas such as waiting rooms or toilets are also kept scrupulously clean.

The main demand of *Standard Precautions* is that every patient must be treated in the same way to satisfy the requirements of discrimination legislation. When HIV/AIDS was first identified many extreme special precautions were taken when treating known sufferers to protect healthcare workers and subsequent patients. This was deemed as discriminatory and *Universal/Standard Precautions* were devised to ensure that cross infection could be minimised or removed but no patient would be treated in a different manner because of their known or unknown infectivity. Hence every patient should be treated in the same way and regarded as being potentially infectious. This also protects healthcare workers and subsequent patients from infection from a patient who does not declare or does not know that they have or are carrying an infection.

Apart from ensuring that your immunity is up to date and appropriate, and that both you and your establishment follow *Standard Precautions,* you should also use PPE and ensure that you follow effective hand hygiene regimes throughout all aspects of your work.

Other considerations for your protection include:

- Wear low heeled or flat shoes that cover the whole of the front of the foot.
- Hair should be tied back so that it cannot fall over the face during chairside work.

- Any religious headwear should be washed daily and tied in such a way as to not interfere with chairside duties.

## What Personal Protective Equipment (PPE) should I use?

There are certain basic items of PPE that you should routinely wear at the chairside and others that you should use for cleaning, decontamination and sterilisation duties. These are outlined below.

### Chairside working

#### 1. Examination gloves
These must be well fitted to allow tactile efficiency. They should also have a roughened surface on the finger tips. Ideally they should be latex free but should not be made of vinyl. Vinyl gloves do not offer sufficient protection at chair-side. It is imperative that the gloves you use routinely fit very well to allow manual dexterity and tactile sensitivity. The gloves must be changed between patients and must be removed before touching any item that cannot be decontaminated effectively, if they are contaminated. They must never be washed or sanitised with alcohol gel. Sterile gloves in individual sizes and packed in single pairs must be worn for surgical procedures.

#### 2. Face masks
Face masks protect you from inhaling contaminated aerosols. There are many types available but the minimum standard must be that the mask is type II filtration and water repellent. It is possible to buy masks which have an integral microbial filter which give increased protection. However this type of mask is more expensive. This type II filtration mask is not adequate for protection if treating a known 'swine flu' case, when a specifically fitted respirator mask must be worn. Some masks have integral eye protection but users must ensure adequate protection is achieved. If these are used it is also possible to purchase face visors but these do not give adequate aerosol protection and a mask should be worn as well. Whatever type of protective mask / visor is used, it must be changed between patients. Paper masks must be thrown away. Visors which are not disposable should be disinfected or decontaminated according to the manufacturer's instructions.

### 3. Eye protection

This is essential to protect the eyes from the aerosol created during treatment. Apart from microscopic blood particle, it will also contain tooth debris or calculus. Apart from the aerosol, other particles can be expelled from the mouth during cavity preparation or scaling. Eye protection should, ideally, be close fitting and wrap around to protect effectively. If you wear prescription glasses routinely, then, depending on the size of the lenses, you may need to wear wrap around protective glasses over the top. Whatever type of eye protection is used it must be thoroughly decontaminated between patients, if it is not disposable or capable of being sterilised. It is also imperative that the eye protection you use is suitable for you. It cannot be a case of 'one size fits all' in the practice.

### 4. Uniform protection

It is becoming more usual for some type of disposable gown or apron to be worn to protect your uniform. Your uniform should not be worn outside the practice, but a disposable apron or gown will reduce the amount of contamination on your uniform. Some type of disposable cover should be worn whenever there is the possibility of blood contamination, i.e. during surgical procedures, extractions, deep scaling etc. As with other PPE, these gowns or aprons must be disposed of between patients and must never be worn from one patient to another.

## Decontamination, sterilising and cleaning

### 1. Examination gloves

For cleaning and decontamination, heavy duty gloves must be worn, which are washed and dried after use and disposed of regularly. Examination gloves should be worn when removing items from the autoclave and bagging.

### 2. Face masks

Should be worn during decontamination procedures and cleaning of equipment such as suction tubings. They are not usually necessary when carrying out general cleaning or taking items from the steriliser although they could be worn if you feel it necessary.

### 3. Eye protection
Essential when carrying out decontamination of equipment or instruments but not essential when for general cleaning or removing items from the steriliser.

### 4. Disposable aprons or gowns
These should be worn for decontamination and general cleaning but not for removing items from the steriliser.

## How do I ensure I effectively wash my hands?

There is a recognised eight stage process for ensuring effective hand hygiene as shown in *Figure 4.2*.

It is possible that the Infection Control Team (ICT) at your local Primary Care Trust (PCT) may be able to come into your practice to demonstrate an effective procedure and test your technique using an Ultra Violet Light Box.

It is a good idea to have a copy of the procedure presented in *Figure 4.2* fixed by every hand wash sink. It is also essential that sinks are designated as either 'Hand wash only' or 'Decontamination only'. It is imperative that the distinction is made and decontamination is not carried out in the same sink as hands are washed.

## When should I wash my hands?

There are some essential times when you should follow the hand wash protocol but it would be better if you get used to always using an effective hand wash technique. It will become second nature in just the same way as basic aspects of your day to day job. You should also be aware that this is important at home as well as at work.

In general, you should wash your hands:

1. **At work**
   - After you have used the toilet.
   - When you first enter the treatment area.
   - Before putting on gloves.
   - After changing from heavy duty to examination gloves.

*Preventing cross infection*

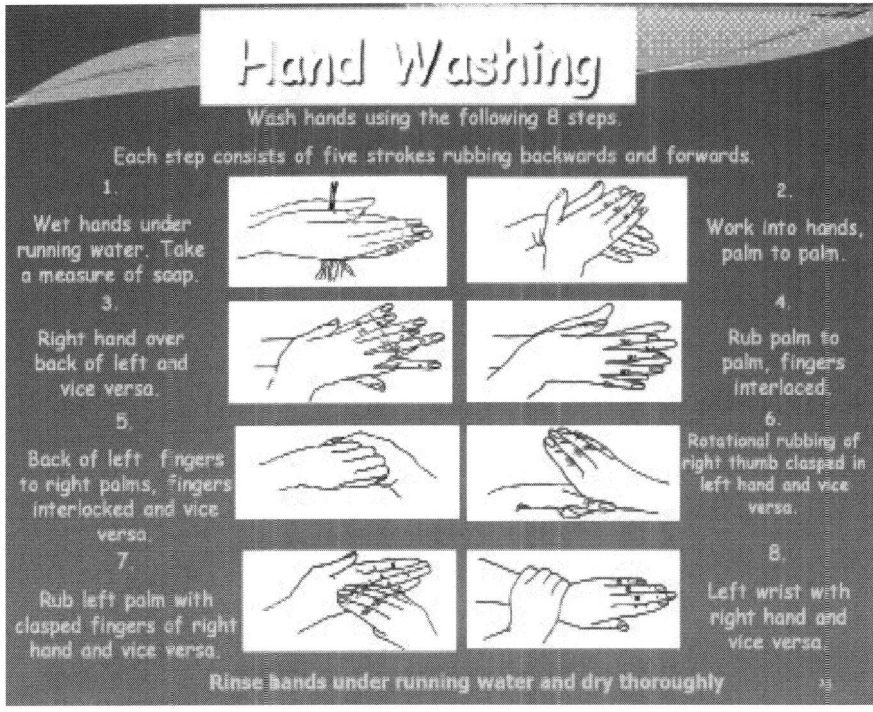

Figure 4.2 Hand washing procedure.

- After taking off gloves.
- After removing PPE.
- When you leave the treatment area.

2. **At home**
   - After using the toilet.
   - After changing a nappy.
   - After cleaning up vomit, faeces or urine.
   - After handling pets.
   - Before handling food.
   - When preparing food between handling raw and cooked food and between preparing meat or vegetables.
   - After finishing cleaning.

## How else can I ensure I carry out effective hand hygiene?

There are other rules that should govern your dress to ensure effective hand hygiene can be achieved.

1. Keep nails short, no nail extensions, and free from varnish or polish or other nail adornments.
2. Do not wear a wrist watch.
3. Only wear a plain wedding band, no costume or stoned rings. Any engagement rings or stoned wedding bands should be covered with tape if they cannot be removed.
4. Wear short sleeves and have disposable arm covers if sleeves cannot be short for religious reasons.
5. Do not wear any wrist adornments. Friendship or religious wrist ornaments should be pushed up the arm and covered with tape.

## Is my personal hygiene important?

It is important that your personal hygiene is impeccable to protect yourself and others in your family. You should shower or take a bath daily and wash your hair as often as possible.

You have taken many precautions to protect yourself in the workplace but the aerosol created during treatment will contaminate you and everything you wear as well as your skin, so personal hygiene and effective laundry techniques are imperative.

It is almost inevitable that you will find that your hands will become dry because of the number of times you will wash them, so careful drying and the use of a good hand cream as often as possible is essential. It is possible to reduce the amount of times you wash your hands by the use of alcohol gels or hand sanitizers. These must not be used in place of washing but only if the hands are visibly clean. Constant use will leave a film on the hands which will encourage bacteria and not help the condition of the skin on your hands.

It is important to keep any scratches or abrasions covered with a waterproof dressing before putting on gloves, if they are on your hands, and covered if on the arms. The aerosol that is produced contains bacteria which, if it gets into an open wound, could lead to an infection and mean that you cannot work until it is clear.

*Preventing cross infection*

## What should I do if I have a 'sharps' injury?

A sharps injury is any injury caused by a sharp, contaminated instrument. This includes used needles, used burs, used matrix bands, airscaler tips or other sharp instruments. It can also include splashes into the mouth or eyes from contaminated liquids or bites from patients.

You must take any such injury very seriously. It is this type of injury that can put you at risk of contacting a blood-borne infection. If you sustain an injury from a contaminated 'sharps' you should:

1. Wash the wound and make it bleed, if possible.
2. Apply a waterproof dressing.
3. Check the patient's medical history to see if they have a known infection.
4. Report in the Practice Accident Book and to the Senior Nurse or Practice Manager.
5. Inform the OHD that you deal with to have your immunity level checked.
6. If there is a doubt about a patient's medical history then you should report to the local Accident and Emergency Department (A&E) for expert medical advice and possible blood tests. Details of the patient's medical history should accompany you to A&E.
7. If the patient has a known blood-borne infection then immediate transfer to A and E is essential.

If you work in a large establishment such as a hospital or in the Personal Dental Service, there will be an agreed protocol to follow which may involve taking blood samples from both donor (patient) and recipient (you).

If you are splashed in the eyes or mouth you should wash the areas with copious amounts of clean, preferably sterile, water. It is important that eyes are flushed very thoroughly and if any doubt about whether there is any debris in the eye, then you should seek immediate medical advice. An antiseptic mouthwash could be taken after rinsing with water.

If you receive a bite from a patient, then the sharps injury procedure described above should be followed.

## Who else can I rely on to protect me?

Basically you must take all sensible precautions to protect yourself and that must be your responsibility. You cannot rely on anyone else to protect you, however, as part of a team, you should make sure that all team members take responsibility to protect themselves so that no-one person puts the others at risk by their actions.

Your employer has a duty of care to make the working environment as safe as is reasonably practical, under the Health and Safety at Work Act 1974. You also have a similar duty of care to work in a way that does not put others at risk.

It is also the case that if you are expected to use gloves on more than one patient or are expected to reuse any single use or disposable item or are not allowed to use appropriate and effective PPE, then you must report it. If the situation does not improve then it must be reported to the GDC because it could put a patient at risk. This is part of your responsibility as a registered dental care professional.

The PPE that is provided for your use must be appropriate and adequate for your needs. This is also a legal requirement under the Personal Protective Equipment at Work Regulations 1992. If the PPE is not adequate and appropriate then the practice owner is liable under these regulations.

The correct PPE must not be governed by the cost but by its adequacy and appropriateness. It must fit well, be of the correct type and be fit for purpose.

A more detailed description of infection control and decontamination and your role and responsibilities can be found in the book *The Dental Nurses Guide to Infection Control and Decontamination* (Porter K 2008).

## References:

British Dental Association (2003) *Advice Sheet A12 – Infection Control in General Dental Practice*

Department of Health (2008) *Health Technical Memorandum 01-05 – Decontamination in Primary Dental Care*

Porter K (2008) *The Dental Nurses Guide to Infection Control and Decontamination* Quay Books, London

# CHAPTER 5

# Radiography

- **Is there a qualification that I need to achieve to take radiographs?**
- **What are the laws and rules on radiography that I should know about?**
- **What should I do if my dentist wants me to do radiographs and I do not have the qualification?**
- **Do I need to learn about radiography for my CPD?**
- **What should I do to assist in the taking of radiographs?**
- **How do I process radiographs?**
- **How do I deal with processing chemicals and film debris safely?**
- **What is digital radiography?**
- **What are the infection prevention and control measures required with regard to radiography?**

## Is there a qualification that I need to achieve to take radiographs?

In 2005 a radiography course accredited by the National Examining Board for Dental Nurses (NEBDN) was launched to allow dental nurses to be taught how to safely take radiographs. The course was developed with the help of the Royal College of Radiographers and the British Society of Dental and Maxillofacial Radiology and supported by the Dental Nurses Standards and Training Advisory Board (DNSTAB) of the General Dental Council (GDC). The course sets out to train dental nurses in both the theory and practice of taking radiographs. Candidates are required to complete a log book of a number of differing radiographs taken as well as a written examination. There are a number of centres accredited to carry out the training, a list of which is available from the National Examining Board for Dental Nurses (NEBDN).

The need for such training was evident when the Ionising Radiation (Medical Exposure) Regulations 2000 (IRMER) was enacted which

51

updated and refined the primary legislation, Ionising Radiation Regulation 1999. This legislation describes the different responsibilities for all practitioners and operators of radiographs. Dental nurses are designated as operators and the legislation demands that all operators who are directly involved in X-raying patients must be adequately trained. This adequate training involves learning theory and developing the practical skills needed to safely carry out dental radiography and comply with the legislation.

Further details of the full curriculum and entrance requirements for this post qualification certificate are available from the NEBDN. The course is only open to registered and qualified dental nurses who have the full support of their dentists. The dentist will have to agree to supervise the trainee and fill in the log book. There is a fee to take this course which will vary depending on the institution that runs it. You cannot expect your dentist to pay this fee for you although some will and some will offer to help by paying part of it. You may also have to obtain agreement from the dentist for time off to attend lectures etc. All this must be taken into account when deciding whether or not to enrol on a course.

## What are the laws and rules on radiography that I should know about?

The rules concerning the taking of radiographs are contained in three pieces of legislation:

1. The Ionising Radiation Regulations 1999 (IRR 1999)
This long document sets out many regulations under the headings:

- Interpretation.
- General principles and procedures.
- Arrangements for the management of radiation protection.
- Designated areas.
- Classification and monitoring of persons.
- Arrangements for the control of radioactive substances, articles and equipment.
- Duties of employees.
- Miscellaneous.

There are also nine other Schedules included in the regulations.

2. The Ionising Radiation (Medical Exposure) Regulations 2000 (IRMER 2000)

This piece of legislation sought to clarify parts of the earlier document and set out more precise regulations on radiography training. It provided a more exact definition and explanation of what is acceptable as 'Adequate Training'. The IRMER 2000 regulations updated the 'local rules' that must be followed in any establishment where radiographs are routinely and regularly taken. These 'local rules' must be written, reviewed and updated regularly, a process which is the responsibility of the dentist in charge of the practice or a designated person, in a larger establishment. If you have the radiography qualification you must comply with these rules and keep up to date with any changes. However you are not and cannot be responsible for compiling or updating them in your practice, but you should prompt the responsible person to update them if you feel this is necessary.

3. The Ionising Radiation Regulations 2004

This legislation updated the laws and regulations to meet current EU directives in this area.

More details on the exact contents of these three pieces of legislation can be found on the website www.legislation.gov.uk.

It is advisable to regularly check on the latest legislation because all legislation is under constant review and revision and is often updated as new directives are agreed by the European Union.

## What should I do if my dentist wants me to do radiographs and I do not have the qualification?

Prior to the introduction of the post qualification certificate in 2005, it was common for dentists in practice to 'train' nurses to take radiographs. At that time neither the dentist or the nurse were actually breaking the law but by taking radiographs without adequate training placed both themselves and their patients at potential risk.

Since the introduction of the qualification, it is now illegal for a dental nurse who is not 'adequately trained' to take radiographs. That 'adequate training' is the achievement of the post qualification certificate.

If your dentist tells you to take radiographs and you do not have the qualification, you must refuse. If you go ahead and a problem arises you will be putting your registration at risk because you will be working outside you *Scope of Practice for Dental Nurses* (GDC 2008).

If your dentist offers to train you but will not support you to take the qualification, then you should also refuse. The training provided would not be deemed as 'adequate' in the terms of the legislation and you could be reported to the GDC.

## Do I need to learn about radiography for my CPD?

Radiography is one of the core subjects and requires annual verifiable updates. The requirement is for 5 hours of verifiable CPD in every 5 year cycle. In other words 1 hour per year every year. Due to the nature of the subject it is important that this CPD is carried out every year and not done in one lump in year one and never touched again.

Dental nurses who have successfully completed the post qualification certificate must also complete an annual update under the IRMER 2000 regulations. This must also be documented. Failure to carry out this update will mean that you cannot legally take radiographs.

## What should I do to assist in the taking of radiographs?

If you do not hold the qualification then you can only assist the person taking the radiograph. You cannot place the film in the mouth or prepare the patient for extra-oral radiographs apart from putting on any protective clothing, i.e thyroid collar etc.

If the radiography machine is in a separate room, then you should accompany the patient to the room, taking the time to check that they fully understand what is going to happen and answering any queries they may have, within your scope of knowledge. You can seat them in the chair and put on the protective clothing, or place them by the machine for taking Orthopantomogram (OPT) radiographs.

Most radiographs taken are intra-oral radiographs (inside the mouth). This means that the film is placed in the patient's mouth and either supported by a specially designed holder or the patient's finger. These radiographs are routinely used to diagnose caries, bone loss or apical condition of teeth.

*Radiography*

An OPT is an extra-oral radiograph (outside the mouth). The film is housed in a holder that is part of a machine which moves around the patient's face to record all the teeth in one long radiograph. For this radiograph to be taken, the patient has to stand inside the machine. This type of radiograph is used as a basic diagnostic tool to look for retained roots, unerupted teeth and other abnormalities. There are other types of extra-oral radiographs which can be used but only on an occasional basis and for very specific diagnoses. These radiograph films are housed in a light proof cassette and require specialist rooms for processing. They can be used for diagnosing disease in the sinus's and for planning orthodontic treatment. These require the patient to stand and be positioned alongside the cassette.

Once the patient has been placed, basically the radiograph taker will fine tune the positioning of the patient in relation to the machine and film. You must then ensure you provide the correct film and the correct holder. Again this will be checked by the taker prior to taking the radiograph and they will place the holder and film in the patient's mouth for intra-oral films. You must not do this, even with supervision, if you are not qualified or still under training.

When the film has been placed, you and the taker should retire behind a screen if provided or should retreat to the furthest extent of the activation buttons cable. The taker should activate the machine. Without qualification you should not activate the machine as this is deemed to be taking the radiograph and outside your scope of practice. The activation of the machine is only to be carried out by someone who is adequately trained under the terms of the IRMER 2000 regulations.

After removing any protective items, you should then accompany the patient back to the treatment area. It is your responsibility to ensure that the equipment is decontaminated ready for subsequent patients and then to process the radiograph.

## How do I process radiographs?

### Extra-oral radiographs

Any extra-oral radiographs must be processed in an automatic processing machine. Cassette and OPT radiographs need to be handled in a light proof room. They need to be opened, the film taken out and then placed in the processor. A fresh film should be put into the cassette and then the cassette closed. The film will come out of the processor dry and can be labelled with the patient's name and the date so that it can be suitably filed after viewing.

### Intra-oral films

These films can be processed either manually or in a processor. Although rare now, you should be aware of how radiographs are processed manually. It is also possible to use 'instant' radiographs which come in a packet which contain the chemicals and which develop the film prior to removing it from the packet. These films do not have the longevity of normally processed films and should only be used in exceptional circumstances.

#### Manual processing

This must be carried out in a light proof area. The room used should have a 'safelight' fitted. This is a light that emits sufficient light to be able to see what you are doing but not enough to affect adversely the image on the film. This light is usually a redish orange colour.

*Process*
1. Put on safelight and unwrap film and place on a hanger. Take care not to handle the film other than at the edges. Careless handling can adversely affect the finished film.
2. Place hanger into the tank containing developer for the recommended time, usually about 1 minute.
3. Remove from developer and shake off excess.
4. Wash in clean water for 30 seconds and shake off excess.
5. Place in tank containing fixer for recommended time, again usually 1 minute.
6. Take out of tank and shake off excess. The safelight can now be turned off and the normal light put on.
7. Wash under running water for at least 1 minute.
8. Check quality and move on hanger to ensure no important area is covered by the hook on the holder. Take care not to handle the middle of the film in its wet state as this can leave marks on the film.

*Radiography*

9. Once viewed it will need to be dried thoroughly prior to being labelled and stored appropriately. This should ideally be overnight.

### Automatic processing

This is carried out in a machine which carries the whole of the previous process automatically and produces a dry film ready for labelling and storage after viewing. It does this with a system of belts that slowly move round in each tank of developer, water, fixer and drier. The belt carries the film through each tank and then passes it on to the next belt and next tank. The big advantage of this system is that you can be doing something else while the film is processed and the film emerges dry and easier to handle, view and store immediately.

*Process*
1. Ensure the machine is turned on early in the morning as they can take time to warm up and be ready for use.
2. Put hands inside machine via the two hand holes. These give access to a lightproof chamber for unwrapping the film.
3. Unwrap the film and feed it into the machine via a slot.
4. Activate the machine and check that the film has fed into the slot completely and been taken into the machine.
5. Remove hands from the holes bringing debris with you.
6. The radiograph will appear at the other end after about 4 – 5 minutes, completely processed and dry.
7. The film can be labelled, checked and stored appropriately.

## How do I deal with processing chemicals and film debris safely?

Whichever way you process the films, the chemicals used must be dealt with carefully and disposed of safely. The chemicals used react with chemicals on the surface of the film which are activated by the X-rays hitting them and all together they produce an image of the structures. Denser structures, i.e. bone, tooth etc will stop most of the X-rays passing through them and will appear white on the film. Where there are no structures present the X-rays will pass straight through appearing black on the film. These structures will appear in varying shades of grey depending on the density of the structure. Tooth enamel will appear solid white whereas bone will be a mottled white where it is less dense.

The processing chemicals used are potentially dangerous and must be handled with care, training in their use is essential and there should be Control of Substances Hazardous to Health Regulations (COSHH) assessments done and available at point of use. These assessments must be regularly reviewed and updated.

The manufacturers of both developer and fixer will provide instructions for their safe use and these must be followed at all times. They will also provide information about safe disposal, again these must be followed at all times. The chemicals need to be changed regularly and this will normally relate to the number of films processed or weekly, again as per the manufacturers instructions. When changing the chemicals, PPE must be worn i.e. gloves, mask, eye protection and disposable aprons. This applies to both manual and mechanical processing as the chemicals used in both are similar.

The spent chemicals after changing must not be disposed of down the sink. They must be collected in separate containers and disposed of by a specialist waste disposal company. Safe disposal of the chemicals is not the only special disposal concerned with radiography. The film packet contains a piece of lead foil which helps to prevent the scatter of the X-rays. This lead foil cannot be disposed of in the clinical waste, it must be stored and disposed of by specialist waste disposal companies. The outer packet and paper inside the film packet can be disposed of in clinical waste.

## What is digital radiography?

The increased use of computerised record keeping in most dental practices created a demand for a way to record radiographs that could also be kept with the patient records on the computer. This brought about digital radiography.

Digital radiographs use the same films as analogue radiographs but instead of the image being produced by the action of chemicals on the film, the image appears on a computer monitor, digitally created from the film. Instead of the film being held in the mouth by a holder, the film is put

*Radiography*

into a specially designed holder that is linked to the computer. The holder contains a sensor which picks up the X-rays after they have passed through the film and digitally reproduces them onto the monitor. The image is then saved within the computer and can be recalled at any time.

The use of digital radiographs makes it much easier to send radiographs to consultants if a patient is referred for specialist advice. They can be sent via email but can also be printed and sent as a hard copy, or downloaded onto a CD that can be sent with the referral letter.

You will assist in a similar way as to normal radiographs as the equipment used is the same, the only slight difference being in the holder used in the mouth.

## What are the Infection Prevention and Control (IPC) measures required with regard to radiography?

It is important that the radiographic equipment of whatever type is thoroughly decontaminated and sterilised. This is particularly important if radiographs are taken during surgical procedures as equipment will be contaminated with blood. It is also important that there is no chance of a patient who has open wounds being contaminated from previous patients. Below is a list of the procedures for decontaminating radiographic equipment:

### Large equipment – machine, processor etc
- The radiography machine and processor must be cleaned in accordance with the manufacturer's instructions. You must fully comply with these instructions as this may lead to the failure of the equipment or to the equipment becoming dangerous to use. You must not cut corners. These pieces of equipment must be maintained regularly and by expert mechanics.
- At the start of the day, cleaning and preparing these pieces of equipment must form part of your regular decontamination regime.
- After each use it should be wiped down thoroughly, particularly parts that have been touched by contaminated gloves, using an appropriate disinfectant.

### Radiography holders
- Any radiography holders must be thoroughly decontaminated in

an ultrasonic bath or washer/disinfector prior to sterilisation. It is not appropriate to only wipe them or soak them in some form of decontaminant, unless this is stated in the manufacturer's instructions.

As with any other decontamination procedure, you should wear appropriate protective clothing. New film packets have an outside cover which is impermeable and protects the inner packet from saliva and also the film inside which can be adversely affected if contaminated with saliva. This outer cover can be torn off and the inner packet handled without contaminating your gloves. This means that you can process the film without changing your gloves and will not contaminate the film.

The chemicals used in processing will decontaminate the film but once they have been processed, they are very easily contaminated by careless handling with contaminated gloves.

Care should be taken when decontaminating digital holders and manufacturer's instructions must be very carefully followed. Using digital radiographs overcomes the problems of possible contamination after processing as they are stored and viewed on the computer.

## References

General Dental Council (2008) *Scope of Practice for Dental Nurses*

# CHAPTER 6

# Role in the care of patients during treatment

- **What is my basic role during any treatment?**
- **What are the basics I should know about mixing materials?**
- **What if the practice is computerised?**
- **What is my role in arranging payments and ensuring forms are correctly filled in?**
- **What is my role in specific treatment?**
  - **New patient assessments**
  - **Filling appointment**
  - **Crown/bridge/onlay appointments**
  - **Denture appointments**
  - **Endodontic appointments**
  - **Orthodontic appointments**
  - **Treating children**
  - **Periodontal appointments**
  - **Sedated patients**
  - **Extractions**
  - **Surgical procedures**
  - **Suture removal/review appointments**
  - **Implant appointments**
  - **Periodontal surgery appointments**
  - **Biopsy appointments**

In this chapter there are suggestions as to your role in preparing the surgery and caring for the patient during the different types of treatment. There are no lists of instruments for each procedure as every dentist has their own preferences and it would be impossible to list all available for any procedure. Your dentist will try out new materials and instruments from time to time as research uncovers new ways of completing a task and new and improved materials to achieve this. There is a responsibility on both you and your dentist to discuss these improvements and agree how you should both proceed.

You should take this as part of your continuing professional development (CDP). CPD is what it says – Continuing Professional Development, a process of continually updating your knowledge and skills and applying them to your everyday job. Dentistry will never stand still and will continually evolve as research introduces new materials, techniques and knowledge. You must take these changes on board.

You will learn your dentist's preferences over a period of time. The lists that follow are only meant as an aide memoire for procedures that you may not assist with very frequently. There are no set right ways to 'nurse' your patient and you will evolve ways that you find you are most comfortable with and that your dentist and the patient is happy with. Your objective must be that the patient has been 'nursed' and cared for competently and is happy at the end of the treatment. If this is achieved then however you have achieved this, it is right approach.

Your techniques will evolve over time as your experience grows. Never be afraid to talk to other more experienced colleagues about how they deal with situations that you have found difficult and learn from them. Remember that you have knowledge that could help them, so they should learn from you also.

## What is my basic role during any treatment?

In very basic terms, your role when patients are being treated is to 'nurse' the patient, i.e. care for the patient and ensure the experience is as pleasant as possible. You have to assist the dentist by providing the instruments they need, preparing and delivering any materials and medicaments needed and working efficiently to ensure the treatment is carried out efficiently and to the highest possible standard.

You have to balance your skills between aspirating water from the patient's mouth, being ready for what the dentist may need next and keeping an eye on the patient's overall comfort and well being. The dentist will be concentrating on what they are doing in the patient's mouth, you have to monitor the patient's overall welfare and notice signs of discomfort or oncoming illness.

The basic things that you should do irrespective of what treatment is being carried out are:

*Role in the care of patients during treatment*

- Collect your patient and take them to the treatment room.
- Chat to the patient to put them at ease.
- Ease them in the chair and put on protective clothing, bib and goggles.
- Note anything in the patient's records that the dentist dictates.
- Listen while the dentist works to get prewarning of what they will be doing and prepare for that.
- Answer any queries for the patient to the depth of your knowledge or refer back to the dentist if unsure.
- Keep the work area tidy and clear away unnecessary items.
- Monitor patient's comfort throughout and alert the dentist if a problem arises.
- When the treatment is complete, take the patient to reception area or where admin is carried out so the patient can make a new appointment or sign any forms.
- Check the patient is content before leaving them.

Practices vary and some may like the receptionist to take the patient to the treatment room. This should be explained to you when you first start. As your experience grows, you should feel comfortable enough to suggest changes in procedures, if you feel that it would improve the patient experience.

## What are the basics I should know about mixing materials?

There are so many different mixing materials that are used in dental treatment that it would need a separate book to list them all and the techniques required for mixing them. It is also a fact that new materials are being introduced and updated versions of old materials brought out all the time, so such a book would be out of date before it was published.

You should get to know all the representatives from the different manufacturers and suppliers and encourage them to come in to explain new materials etc at regular intervals. This is another opportunity for CPD collection. Most reps will be only too happy to come into a practice to demonstrate new materials and techniques; after all this is their job. If the dentist attends a meeting and comes back with new ideas and materials, suggest that you arrange for the relevant rep to come in and demonstrate it to everyone in the practice. After all, the dentist will use it but you have to mix it and present it correctly for it to work properly. You will also need to understand how much stock is required so that it doesn't go out of date and how it is best maintained.

In general, always read carefully and understand the manufacturer's instructions prior to first using it on a patient. The following is a guide on how to mix your materials:

### Powder and liquid materials
- Always use the measures that are provided. If no measures are provided, check the instructions as to proportions of powder to liquid.
- Mix it to the manufacturer's instructions on the advised pad or glass slab.
- Never put the spatula into the bottle of powder to remove some powder, this will contaminate the remaining powder.
- Check use-by dates regularly.
- Always put lid back onto bottles immediately.
- Mix it to the required thickness for the dentist's needs.
- For alginate materials, always shake the powder prior to measuring out.
- Always use clean glass slabs and spatulas or paper pads.
- Remove mixed material from spatula and from instruments as soon as possible, preferably before it sets.

### Impression materials
- Make sure you have everything you need for the impression to be taken. Putty/heavy bodied, light bodied or wash, syringe tips, mixing tips depending on the type of material used.
- Have a range of impression trays available.
- Make sure you have enough material for the impression.
- Put everything ready and to hand on a paper towel.
- Ensure the spatula you use, if using one, is clean.
- Take care not to contaminate any containers, cartridge syringes etc.
- Put caps back onto tubes, lids onto pots etc, immediately and carefully, taking care to put correct tops onto correct tubes, tubs etc.
- Listen to what the dentist says and act on their instructions.
- Have disinfectants available to disinfect impressions after taken.

### Two paste materials
- Any material supplied in two pastes are usually mixed on paper pads.
- Put out equal lengths of each paste.
- Put tops back onto correct tubes immediately.
- Mix the pastes together.
- Hand to dentist.
- Wipe spatula clean and wipe any instruments used.

## What if the practice is computerised?

If you routinely work with computerised treatment records, you will not require paper charts to fill in or paper records to write treatments on, all these records will be entered directly into the computer. There are many different computer software packages available which are upgraded constantly so you must learn what your practice uses and be completely happy with working with the package before starting to work unsupervised

Remember that you cannot be working efficiently at the chairside and caring for the patient if you are also expected to enter records into the computer at the same time. The only thing you can do when the dentist is actually treating the patient is record the initial charting. It is essential that chartings, whether computer or manually recorded are inputted accurately. You must listen carefully and query any call that you are not sure of. Again, you will learn with experience of working with one dentist all the time, just how they like to call a charting.

Remember when you are using the computer to take extreme care not to contaminate the keyboard, mouse etc. Always ensure you have clean gloves or washed, ungloved hands when you are using the computer.

## What is my role in arranging payments and ensuring forms are correctly filled in?

This will depend very much on how your practice is set up and administered. In some practices you will be expected to get the patient to fill in all the necessary forms and accept payments. You may also have some responsibility for banking money and recording payments for accounts.

In other practices this will be undertaken by the practice manager or the reception staff or a combination of the two. This must be explained to you when you first join the practice and you must be completely happy with what you have to do. If any of the forms are incorrectly completed this could result in payments not being made or misunderstandings happening. You must also be satisfied that you can explain the forms and the need for them to the patients and answer any questions they have.

## What is my role in specific treatment?

Whatever the treatment is that is being carried out, you must always ensure that both you and your patient has and wears the appropriate protective equipment. Below are some guidelines for specific procedures.

### New patient assessments

You have a prime role in impressing the patient with how the practice looks after its patients. For this treatment you should:

- Meet the patient, introduce both yourself and the dentist. Try to find out a little about them so that you can be more personal with them. Find out how they prefer to be addressed, by their title or by their first name.
- Have all necessary instruments available.
- Make sure the patient is seated comfortably. Put on the protective items and explain the need for their use. If the patient is elderly or infirm, check if they are able to lie flat for treatment and alert the dentist if there is a problem in this area.
- Be prepared to make notes either on their paper record or into the computer, particularly the basic charting. You may have to record a medical history and be prepared to answer questions from the patient.
- Take the patient to the X-ray room and assist whilst any radiographs are taken. Process the radiographs and present to the dentist.
- Make sure that the patient understands what the dentist is advising.
- Take the patient to the person who administers the forms and payments and explain what needs to be arranged .

*Role in the care of patients during treatment*

- Always check that the patient is happy with what has been agreed and discharge them.
- Check if they have any further queries and arrange a further appointment if necessary.

### Filling appointments

This type of treatment is the 'bread and butter' for most general dental practitioners. The fillings provided could be either silver (amalgam) or white (composite), each of which require different specialist equipment for the mixing, placement and setting of the material. For this treatment you should:

- Welcome the patient and seat them. Put on the protective items.
- Have all the instruments and materials at hand, as well as any relevant radiographs and chartings available.
- Support the patient during the giving of the local anaesthetic.
- Monitor the patient for signs of distress.
- Aspirate the mouth while the dentist prepares the cavity, ensuring you keep the working field clear and that you do not obstruct the dentist whilst working.
- Prepare any lining materials as necessary and hand to the dentist.
- Wipe clean any instruments and the spatula you have used.
- Prepare the filling material, either amalgam or composite.
- If amalgam, have the mixer switched on. If composite, have the light curing machine and the necessary etch and bond. The dentist may also wish to place a rubber dam for either filling. Have the instruments and dam ready.
- Assist the dentist whilst the filling is placed, aspirating any excess amalgam or timing the light curing of composite material and providing effective shielding for the patient from the UV light.
- Assist whilst the filling is finished providing articulating paper etc to check that the filling is not high in the occlusion.
- Monitor the patient throughout either procedure.
- Discharge the patient, checking they are happy with what has been done and showing the patient the filling, if they wish to see it.
- Clear up and prepare for the next patient. Ensure waste amalgam and spent amalgam capsules as well as any sharps are disposed of correctly.

## Crown/bridge/onlay appointments

Your role is very similar to that of a filling appointment. For this treatment you should:

- Ensure the correct impression materials are available, impression trays and disinfectant for decontaminating the impression after it has been taken.
- The appointment will be longer and you will need to monitor the patient for a longer time. Ensure that they completely understand what is being done.
- You may need to put a larger plastic apron onto the patient to prepare for impressions to be taken; this will protect the patient's clothing from any dropped impression material.
- Support the patient while the impressions are taken. It is important that you know if the patient has a bad gag reflex which will cause them to retch and have discomfort while the impressions are in the mouth. Talk to the patient and reassure them. Provide a bowl for them to catch excess saliva. Be prepared to decrease the setting time of materials if possible, using warmer water for the alginate or use extra catalyst to decrease setting time. This can only be done with experience.
- Support the patient during the making of a temporary crown or bridge and mix the appropriate materials.
- For an appointment to fit an indirect restoration, you should have the crown/bridge ready from the laboratory, suitably decontaminated.
- Have the cement and articulating paper ready to check the finished restoration is not high on the bite.
- If a veneer is to be fitted, have the appropriate composite material and all the accessory materials ready.
- Have a mirror handy to show the patient how the finished restoration looks prior to final fitting.
- Aspirate while excess cement is removed.
- Discharge the patient ensuring that they are completely happy and offer a further appointment for a check, if required.
- Clear away and ensure correct disposal of items and decontamination of all the instruments.

### Denture appointments

There could be many appointments involved in the making of a denture or there could be just a couple. This depends on the decision of the dentist. At each appointment there will be materials required and these will have to be disinfected prior to sending to the laboratory. For this treatment you should:

- Reassure the patient at every stage. The patient is liable to be elderly and need careful monitoring and very careful explanations.
- It may be necessary to explain to a carer or escort if an elderly patient is frail or not completely 'with it'. Always talk to the patient first and only address the escort/carer if total understanding cannot be achieved.
- Ensure the patient is comfortable in the chair and that it is not laid flat if the patient is uncomfortable.
- Give support while impressions are taken and clean patient's face afterwards.
- Talk to the patient during times that the dentist is working on wax try-ins etc outside the patient's mouth. Get to know the patient so that you can talk about things relevant to the patient, i.e. grandchildren etc.
- When the denture is actually fitted, ensure the patient understands how to look after it and how they put it into and take it out of the mouth.
- Provide a mirror so that the dentist can demonstrate how to carry out these procedures.
- Give the patient their old dentures back in a bag, where applicable.
- Discharge the patient and ensure they have a further appointment to review the fit of the denture, particularly if it is their first denture.
- Clear the surgery away, ensuring safe disposal of all items and efficient decontamination of instruments. Ensure any impressions or other lab work is disinfected effectively and packaged ready for transfer to the laboratory, along with any appropriate paperwork.

## Endodontic appointments

Endodontics is a field that has changed fundamentally over the past few years and will continue to do so, using more and more mechanical means. You will need to ensure you stay up to date with new developments.

- The materials, instruments etc required will depend on what stage of the endodontics is being carried out. At every stage you will need to have out rubber dam sheets and equipment, endodontic files and medicaments.
- You will need to monitor the patient closely if rubber dam is used as you may have to aspirate under it, if a saliva ejector isn't used.
- You will need to develop a technique for aspiration of water from the handpieces if used when rubber dam is in place. This can only come with experience. You must ensure that the water is effectively aspirated from the rubber dam and that none runs off onto the patient.
- It may be advisable to put a larger plastic apron on the patient to protect them from water run off from the dam, as well as from irrigation solutions used.
- Depending on how the dentist likes to work, they may expect you to provide close support and hand the endodontic files and other small items.
- You will have to closely aspirate the access cavity of the tooth when the canals are irrigated with sodium hypochlorite (bleach), to stop any of the bleach getting into the patients mouth around the rubber dam. There are small bore aspiration tips available to make this easier.
- A radiograph will need to be taken at least once during the whole procedure, or even at every stage. You should have the radiography machine ready, the processor turned on and any holders ready for use.
- If a radiograph was taken at a previous appointment, this should be available for the dentist to consult during treatment.
- At the final stage, obturation, you will need to have filling materials for the canal as well as the access cavity. The canal is usually filled with gutta percha, a plastic material. This can be placed using a 'point' which is a tapered piece of gutta percha which corresponds to the size of the files that were used to clean the canal.

*Role in the care of patients during treatment*

- This is 'cemented' in place using a sealing material usually supplied as two pastes which are mixed together. This cement takes many hours to finally set so that the dentist has sufficient working time to add extra fine points to ensure that the whole canal is filled. This can also be done using a machine which warms the gutta percha and makes it easier to compact into the canal.
- The canal can be prepared using hand files or rotary instruments, this will depend on the preferences of the dentist.
- When the treatment is completed, inside the canal, then the access cavity in the tooth will be filled in a similar way to other fillings.
- The dentist will usually take a radiograph after the treatment is completely to check that the canal has been effectively filled to the apex and that no filling material has gone through the apex of the tooth.
- You should discharge the patient ensuring that they understand what has been done and arrange any future treatment or appointments that are required.
- Clear the surgery ensuring effective decontamination of all surfaces and equipment used and the safe disposal of all sharps and disposable items.

### Orthodontic appointments

Orthodontic treatment is very specialised and will often be undertaken by a dentist who specialises in this type of treatment and sets up the practice to do no other forms of treatment. The instruments used are very specialised as are the other items used to actually perform the treatment which can take many forms. You will need to learn all the specialist instruments and techniques used for the treatment to be carried out effectively.

- Assessment sessions will definitely require radiographs and impressions so you must be prepared for these procedures.
- The patients are often children who will be accompanied by a parent or guardian. You must be sure that both the patient and the parent/guardian understands what is being advised and what treatment is being prescribed. Orthodontic treatment will often take years to be completed and requires commitment from both the patient and parent/guardian to be successful.
- You will need to support the patient during the taking of impressions

and radiographs and ensure the impressions are disinfected effectively and packed ready for transfer to the laboratory with appropriate paperwork.
- When bands and brackets are being fitted, you should have the necessary items available and the appropriate cements or bonding materials, along with the appropriate arch wires, ligatures, power chains etc ready.
- When the treatment session is finished, ensure the patient has any appropriate literature to explain the care of the appliance that has been fitted. Also thoroughly explain the need for good oral health.
- The patient should have a follow up appointment made before they leave and you should be prepared to answer any questions that the patient may have and also be prepared to alert the dentist if the patient has a query that you cannot answer.
- At some stages of some types of treatment, it may be necessary to give the patient power chains that have to be changed at intervals before the next appointment.
- Some appliances need to be adjusted using a small allen key to adjust a small screw which forms part of the appliance. Some will require attachment to a head band.
- It is advisable for the practice, if orthodontic only, to have some pre-prepared leaflets to give to the patient that explains exactly what has been done and what is expected of them between appointments.
- After the patient is discharged, ensure the surgery is cleared and decontaminated effectively, all equipment is decontaminated and sterilised and impressions are dealt with efficiently. Any bands or brackets that have been removed along with unwanted wires etc should be disposed of in a sharps bin.

## *Treating children*

The overriding role that you have is putting the patient at their ease. Your focus must always be on the child being treated. You will have to be prepared to work much more quickly as the patient will not be able to lie still in the chair for long periods of time. You will also have to adjust your techniques for aspiration and mixing materials where more rapid setting is advisable. Your role during treatment is much the same as for

*Role in the care of patients during treatment*

adults and the instruments and medicaments used will be the same.

- When you prepare the surgery, have all the equipment you need to hand but not necessarily on show as this may frighten a nervous child. Be aware that the child's escort may also be nervous of being at the dentist.
- When you talk to the patient don't use jargon or any terminology that could frighten a child, i.e. the words needle or injection.
- If the patient requires a local anaesthetic, prepare it out of sight of the patient and hand to the dentist behind the child so that they don't see it until the last possible moment. It is usual to use a surface anaesthetic paste to numb the gum around the injection site.
- If a child becomes upset then you may have to enlist the help of the accompanying parent or guardian to calm the child. It is advisable to have the parent or guardian present in the surgery when treatment is carried out.
- Be aware of what the parent is saying as they can sometimes frighten a child inadvertently by what they say and could let their own fear of dental treatment be expressed in what they say and how they act.
- It is a good idea to have some stickers to give a child after treatment. You could also have some sheets for colouring in to give to a child, or anything else that makes the experience more enjoyable. Some practices will have tabards that their nurses can wear to make them look less clinical when children are being treated.
- Try to smile all the time to reassure the child, especially if something goes wrong. Get them to tell you all about what they have been doing or what they did on holiday etc, to put them at ease.
- Experience will change your ways of working with children. You will evolve ways of working which will make the patient experience better. If you have problems or feel you could do better, then talk to your more experienced colleagues.

### Periodontal appointments

Periodontal treatment involves the treatment of the gums (gingivae) and other tissues which surround the tooth. This most often involves the removal of hard deposits which form around the teeth at the level of the gum or just below.

- At an assessment appointment you may need to have differing charting forms to record pocket depth and an index of the amount of plaque and bleeding present in the patient's mouth. This assessment will guide the dentist to the best possible treatment. The patient may also need radiographs to assess the amount of bone that has been lost around the teeth.
- You will need to prepare scaling instruments both mechanical and hand. These instruments are shaped to fit round the tooth with a cutting edge which removes the hard deposits. There are different shapes for different teeth and different scalers for removing supra-gingival (above the gum) deposits or sub-gingival (below the gum) deposits.
- You may be required to sharpen these hand scaling instruments. You should ensure that you have adequate and appropriate training in the correct method of doing this. If done incorrectly, the instrument will be unusable.
- The patient will usually have a mouth wash given prior to treatment. You will be asked to give the patient the mouthwash and advise the patient to swish it around the mouth for 1 minute and then spit it out.
- If mechanical scaling is carried out, you will need to aspirate the water from the patient's mouth and it is essential that you wear a mask and goggles during this to protect yourself from the contaminated aerosol that is produced, which will almost certainly contain both blood and particles of calculus (deposit).
- You should monitor the patient throughout the treatment to be aware of pain or discomfort that the patient may be experiencing. Some dentists will routinely give a local anaesthetic when deep scaling is done.
- At the end of treatment you should ensure that the patient is comfortable and given post treatment advice, as prescribed by the dentist.
- Ensure the patient has a further appointment if necessary.
- When the patient has been discharged you must follow a robust regime of decontamination because of the presence of blood contaminated spatter. The instruments must be thoroughly decontaminated and sterilised. Machines that are used for mechanical scaling must be thoroughly decontaminated and the water reservoirs emptied.
- All disposable items must be disposed of effectively in appropriate containers and bags.

*Role in the care of patients during treatment*

### Sedated patients

It must be stated that you should not be the only person assisting with the treatment of sedated patients, if you do not have the post qualification certificate in the treatment of patients under conscious sedation. If your dentist asks you to cover for a colleague who has the qualification, when you do not, you must refuse.

The training to successfully achieve this qualification covers the monitoring of patients using pulse oximeter machines, the preparation of sedation drugs, the preparation of the machine for administering inhalation sedation (relative analgesia) etc. This is all necessary as there is a greater danger to the wellbeing of the patient while being treated under sedation.

If you have the qualification then you will find added responsibilities being given to you. Some dentists will insist on having two nurses present when treating these patients, one as the qualified person and a runner to assist.

The patient has to agree to certain conditions before they can be treated under sedation, depending on the form of sedation taken. Patients being treated under conscious sedation of whatever type, must never be left unattended at any time whilst sedated or until fully recovered.

- If treated under inhalation sedation or relative analgesia, which is a mixture of nitrous oxide and oxygen which the patient inhales and leaves them in a happy state, the patient can go home under their own steam after treatment. This is because all the sedation drugs, the gases, are expelled from the body when the patient is given 100% oxygen at the end of treatment. If intravenous sedation is given, where a sedative is injected into the blood stream, they must be accompanied to get home and must not drive.
- You must ensure that the necessary pre-treatment instructions are given and understood prior to the treatment appointment being given. You should also check that the instructions have been followed prior to the sedation being given. This will usually be checked again by the dentist.
- You must be sure that the emergency equipment is adequate to the type of sedation being administered and that the sedation drugs are kept in the right conditions and in a locked cupboard. You will also be responsible for logging the use of the drugs and that the antidote drugs are available and all kept in date.

- During treatment you must monitor the patient closely, recording blood pressure, pulse and oxygen saturation at intervals and advising the dentist if a problem arises.
- You should reassure the patient constantly and talk to them. They will be able to talk to you throughout treatment and should never completely lose consciousness. The patient will still exhibit fear during the treatment and you must talk them through what is happening and reassure them.
- The patient will still be able react when a local anaesthetic is given and may react to the noise of the drills if that is their major fear. They will, however not remember what has been done to them after the treatment has been finished. The intravenous sedation drugs contain a substance which will mean that they have no memory of what is happening to them for about half an hour after it is given.
- If inhalation sedation is used, you may have to adapt your working positions to accommodate the nose piece which delivers the gases.
- Apart from the higher level of monitoring of the patient, your role during the treatment is much the same as for the same treatment carried out without sedation.
- At the end of the treatment the patient must be fully recovered from the sedation prior to leaving the surgery. With inhalation sedation, the patient should be ready to leave after a short recovery time. With intravenous sedation, the patient must be kept until fully recovered from the intravenous drug which could be half an hour or more, depending on how much drug was given and how long the treatment took. The patient must be accompanied home and must be given very specific post treatment instructions. The dentist should be the one to discharge the patient after sedation.
- After treatment the surgery should be cleared in a similar way to treatment without sedation. In addition, you should record the drugs used and ensure that any extra equipment is decontaminated and put away.

### Extractions

A patient attending for extractions will usually be nervous and apprehensive so when preparing the instruments, it would be advisable to keep them covered so as not to alarm the patient. For this treatment you should:

*Role in the care of patients during treatment*

- Prepare the instruments and paperwork as previously. If there are radiographs available these should be put onto the viewer. The instruments should be covered or at least not in view of the patient until needed.
- Greet the patient and put them at their ease. Check that they are fully aware of what is going to happen and answer any questions they have. You should check that they have had their usual meal prior to the appointment, i e. breakfast or lunch. If not, then consider giving a glucose drink to raise the blood sugar level, if appropriate.
- Seat the patient and put on appropriate protective items.
- Monitor the patient during the administration of the local anaesthetic and offer support. Continue to monitor after the anaesthetic is given. Watch for signs of fainting, pallor, sweating etc.
- Reassure the patient during the extraction procedure, especially when there are cracking noises during the process.
- After the tooth has been extracted, either place or hand the bite pack for the dentist to place. You should check if the patient wants to keep the tooth and wash it and wrap it up if they do.
- The dentist may ask you to check haemostasis (bleeding) has stopped, or may wish to check themselves. Whichever way, once haemostasis is assured you should give the patient the post extraction instructions that have been agreed by the dentist. Wipe any blood from the patient's face and ensure they feel well enough to leave.
- When clearing the surgery, ensure the area and all the instruments are thoroughly decontaminated and sterilised where possible. Ensure all disposable items are disposed of appropriately, including sharps and the extracted tooth.

### *Surgical procedures*

Your role is very much the same as for extractions but there may be a need for the use of sterile covers for the instruments and the wearing of gowns or other covers to protect uniforms from blood spatter.

- You should prepare the instruments by placing them onto a sterile cover and use sterile gloves to perform the procedure. It may be necessary to use different hand pieces which use sterile water from a

separate system. The instruments should be covered until needed, so as not to alarm the patient but to also retain asepsis.
- You must wear full protective equipment including a cover for your uniform.
- You should support the patient while the local anaesthetic is given and throughout the procedure, being particularly aware of the patient becoming faint.
- During the procedure you must keep the working field clear of blood by aspirating closely at the site of work. At the same time you must keep the floor of the mouth free from saliva and blood. The dentist may also ask you to retract tissues using retractors or a mouth mirror.
- You should assist whilst the sutures are placed by aspirating the field and possibly cutting the sutures, depending on what the dentist requires.
- Once the suturing is complete and the procedure finished you should clean the patients face and check that they feel well. You should cover the used instruments as soon as possible so that the patient cannot see them as they recover. You should keep the patient at the practice for a few minutes to ensure the patient is fit to leave.
- You should ensure that the patient has a further appointment for the removal of the sutures and to check the healing.
- Once the dentist is happy that the patient is fully recovered and ready to go home, then the patient can leave. It shouldn't be your responsibility to discharge the patient after a surgical procedure.

### Suture removal/review appointments

When greeting these patients, enquire as to their experience following the surgery to find out if they have had problems with swelling or discomfort after more than a couple of days. Any problems which they report should be reported to the dentist.

- You should prepare the surgery with instruments to remove the sutures. You should also be prepared for a radiograph to be taken after some surgical procedures to assess healing, i.e. apicectomy or cyst removal.
- You may be asked to remove the sutures yourself but you should only undertake this if you have been trained and only after the dentist

has assessed the patient initially. The dentist will also need to check the patient after the sutures have been removed.
- Whether or not you remove the sutures, the dentist must check the patient prior to discharge and must decide on the need for further appointments or treatment.

### Implant appointments

Implantology is a very specialised and complicated treatment which does not just involve a surgical procedure to place an implant to attach an indirect restoration or denture to. It is not a procedure that is often carried out in general dental practice. It is more often carried out in a dental hospital which specialises in this type of treatment and is very much geared to carry it out and look after the patient.

There are many different types of implant and many ways of fitting them and aftercare will be required. It is essential that before you assist with these types of treatment, you are fully trained and advised by the dentist and by more experienced colleagues.

- There are several stages necessary prior to the actual surgical procedure. The patient must be assessed as to their suitability for the treatment as well as provided counselling to assess the effect on their whole wellbeing if the implant is or is not done.
- They should have radiographs and impressions taken. They should have a session to fully explain exactly what will happen, what the results will be, and what would happen if the implants fail. The patient must agree to keep scrupulous oral hygiene and demonstrate that they can prior to the final decision being taken.
- During these preparatory sessions you must support the patient, offer answers to their questions and support the statements of the dentist. You will need to ensure a sufficient supply of all the many components needed to fit the implant. It is imperative that all the components are sterile and maintained in a sterile state. You must also ensure that there are sufficient supplies of other sterile items, covers, gauze etc.
- On the day of the surgical procedure, you must prepare the surgery with efficient aseptic techniques ensuring sterility is maintained of all

sterile items. You should have all necessary instruments and all the components of the implant kit available and at hand.
- Radiographs should be placed on the viewer.
- When preparing the patient you should answer any questions and put them at their ease as far as possible, making sure that they fully prepared for what is about to happen. You should put on all necessary protective equipment, possibly including sterile covers over their bib.
- During the procedure you should monitor the patient and alert the dentist if there are any problems. You should keep the operating field clear and ensure that all instruments are at hand as they are needed.
- You should assist during the placement of sutures and temporary copings to cover the implants.
- When the procedure is complete, reassure the patient and make them more comfortable. Wipe any blood from the face and answer any questions. The dentist should explain to the patient exactly what has been done and how the procedure has gone.
- You will need to carefully decontaminate all instruments and equipment and sterilise as appropriate. All contaminated sharps must be disposed of appropriately as with all disposable items. It is essential that all non-disposable components of the implant kit are retained, decontaminated and sterilised.
- The patient must be given a further appointment for suture removal and assessment of healing. There will be a series of further appointments to assess healing and check that the patient is maintaining oral hygiene. There will also be assessment of how the implant is embedding into the bone (oseo-integrating).
- After the implant has integrated into the bone and is stable, the final restoration or denture will be made and fitted.

### Periodontal surgery appointments

Your roles and responsibilities are much the same as for other surgical procedures. You will have to prepare mechanical scaling machines and have periodontal packs ready to be mixed.

*Role in the care of patients during treatment*

### Biopsy appointments

Your roles and responsibilities are the same as for other surgical procedures but you must be ready to retrieve the biopsy specimen.

- You will need a pot to put the specimen in and a form to request the investigation to be carried out. You will also be responsible for ensuring that the specimen is packaged appropriately to be sent to the laboratory.
- You should also ensure that the patient has a follow up appointment to have the results of the investigation and any follow up treatment arranged that is necessary. If there is any question that the specimen may be cancerous, the follow up appointment must be as soon as possible after the results are received.
- You must support the patient at the follow up appointment and be ready to answer any questions that they may have.

# CHAPTER 7

# Role in giving patients bad news

- **Should I be the person who gives the patient bad news?**
- **How do I offer the patient support after they receive bad news?**
- **What do I do if the patient asks me questions that I cannot answer?**
- **How should I deal with telephone queries?**
- **What should I do when dealing with a difficult patient?**

## Should I be the person who gives the patient bad news?

It is the responsibility of the dentist to give a patient bad news. This could be a negative test result from a biopsy or radiograph, scan etc. You should never be expected to give a patient such information.

The dentist has the knowledge to answer any questions that the patient has and must be prepared to honestly answer their questions.

Your role is the essential one of providing support and comfort to the patient.

## How do I offer the patient support after they receive bad news?

It is important that you fully understand the situation and what the dentist is about to tell the patient. A lot of this knowledge will come with the experience of working with such cases over a period of time. However much experience you have, you must always be sure of your facts and exactly what support you are expected to give. It would be an advantage to the patient if you and the dentist have discussed what you are about to tell the patient so that you are both prepared for the questions to come.

The dentist will explain the diagnosis and what the treatment options are. Should the patient be diagnosed with a carcinoma or other cancerous lesion, then they may not hear much of what is said after the word 'cancer'. Time must be taken to repeat the information on more than one occasion if necessary.

This is where you must be most supportive. Listen to what is said and observe the reactions of the patient. It could be that the dentist will leave you to support the patient after they have explained the next steps in the treatment regime. It is then that you will need to understand what the dentist has said and meant so that you can answer any questions and explain in simple terms so that they fully understand.

Before you talk to a patient or answer their questions, be sure of the facts of the case and be ready to explain that you need to seek advice if you feel that you cannot deal with the problem. It is better you give accurate advice, even if this means having to obtain that advice and contacting the patient later, rather than give an instant inaccurate answer. If you are accompanying the dentist whilst he talks to the patient, be supportive to the patient, show empathy but never be afraid to tell the truth. It's how you tell this truth that is important.

Ensure the patient fully understands the implications of what they are being told. Be prepared to put jargon into simple terms to ensure understanding. If the dentist has bad news to tell the patient, it is you they will turn to for support and comfort. You must fulfil the difficult task of supporting both the dentist and the patient, this is a skill which truly does come with experience. Do not be tempted to counsel a patient unless you have the training and skills to do so. This is an area that some dental nurses take extra training in to enhance their dental nursing skills. It is also possible to take communication courses to enhance your general communication skills.

## What do I do if the patient asks me questions that I cannot answer?

It is imperative that you do not try to bluff your way out of the situation. You must get the dentist to explain again and keep on until all the patient's questions are answered and that the patient is satisfied. Both you and the dentist must be prepared to spend as much time as it takes with the patient.

It is important that you offer support but not false hope. You must truthfully answer all questions. It is also important that you ensure the patients' and any accompanying relatives' understanding before they leave the surgery. You must be sure that the next step is taken, i.e. letters or phone calls of referral to specialists etc.

## How should I deal with telephone queries?

In general you must be prepared to take the time to answer any queries but if this is over the telephone you must be sure to whom you are talking to. As a general rule you should not discuss any patient's treatment over the telephone. You cannot be sure who you are speaking to, so if someone calls with a query, you should advise them to attend the surgery so that you can talk to them face to face, with a relative present if possible.

You could also receive queries after the patient has been seen by a specialist. This is more difficult and the specialist should give the patient all the time they need to ensure understanding. However you should help if you can as the patient will empathise more easily with you because they know you.

You should remember that, to patients, you are the 'caring face' of dentistry. You are the one they will turn to for help, support and comfort.

## What should I do when dealing with a difficult patient?

Whenever you are talking to a patient, in whatever circumstances, you should always be courteous. Never answer back to them however rude you may think they are being. You must be conscious of religious conventions when directing your questions and/or answers to the patient. If the patient is a minor, then you should direct your communication to the parent or guardian, but do not ignore the child.

If you need to talk to a patient away from the treatment area, in instances of complaint, or confidential conversations, take them to a quiet room where you will not be disturbed and can give the patient your complete attention. You should always listen to the patient, and make it obvious you are listening. Let them have their say. If they are making a complaint, do not interrupt; then answer their queries point by point. If necessary take notes so that you do not forget anything.

If you are confronted by an aggressive patient, do not speak to them in front of a waiting room full of patients. Take them away but ensure you do not put yourself at risk by isolating yourself. If you believe a patient may become violent, then ensure someone else in the practice knows where you are and ensure you can make a speedy escape from any room you take them to. You have the right to refuse to deal with such a patient and insist that the dentist deals with them.

## Sources of further information and guidance

General Dental Council   www.gdc-uk.org
Scope of Practice for Dental Nurses   www.gdc-uk.org
Standards for Dental Professionals   www.gdc-uk.org
British Association of Dental Nurses   www.badn.org.uk
National Examining Board for Dental Nurses   www.nebdn.org

# SECTION 2

# PROFESSIONAL PRACTICE

# CHAPTER 8

# Professional practice requirements and CPD

- **What are the GDC principles of dental practice?**
- **What are the *Standards for Professional Practice*?**
- **What are my obligations regarding equal opportunity?**
- **What are my responsibilities to the patient to ensure they understand what their treatment involves?**
- **What are my responsibilities regarding patient confidentiality?**
- **What are my responsibilities to other members of the team?**
- **What should I do if I feel that the patients are not being treated correctly?**
- **What indemnity insurance do I need to have?**
- **What happens if I am not covered?**
- **What should I do if a claim is made against me?**
- **Why is this important for practice?**
- **What are my obligations regarding CPD?**
- **How can I gain my CPD?**
- **Should my employer provide my CPD?**
- **What further training can I do to further my career?**
- **Should my practice principal keep my GDC registration certificate?**
- **Should my employer employ qualified nurses who are not registered?**

It is not sufficient for you to just qualify to call yourself or work as a 'Dental Nurse'. Since July 2008 it has been illegal to work as a 'Dental Nurse' unless you are registered with the General Dental Council (GDC) and must be renewed annually. If you work as, or call yourself a 'Dental Nurse' and are not registered, you are breaking the law and could be prosecuted, as could any dentist who employs you.

## What are the GDC principles of dental practice?

The GDC sets out six principles within the *Standards for Dental Professionals* (2008). These are:

1. Putting patient's interests first and act to protect them.
2. Respect patient's dignity and choices.
3. Protect the confidentiality of patient's information.
4. Co-operate with other members of the dental team and other healthcare colleagues in the interests of patients.
5. Maintain your professional knowledge and competence.
6. Be trustworthy.

This main booklet is supported by other guidance documents which should be used as principles to work by, not rules to be governed by. These principles are outlined in a booklet which each registrant should have know and understand.

The GDC also produced a series of booklets in 2008 which give guidance for registrants in various aspects such as:

1. Patient confidentiality
2. Team working.
3. Complaints handling.
4. Raising concerns.
5. Management responsibility.

## What are the *Standards for Dental Professionals*?

It is every registrant's responsibility to keep up to date with both the *Standards for Dental Professionals* (2008) and the *Scope of Practice for Dental Nurses (2008)* as issued by the GDC. These are the standards which were devised for all Dental Care Professionals (DCP). They are the standards that must be adhered to in order to maintain your professional status and your registration. The standards are what you will be judged against if a patient makes a complaint against you and these are the standards you will have to defend your actions against. Some of the main clauses from the *Standards for Dental Professionals* (GDC 2008) are discussed next.

- *1.3. Work within your knowledge, professional competence and physical abilities; refer patients for a second opinion for further advice.*

This means that you should not take on any duties for which you have not been trained and which you feel uncomfortable about completing. See also Chapter 3 for discussion on *Scope of Practice for Dental Nurse*.

- *5.4. Find out about laws and regulations which affect your work, premises, equipment and business and follow them.*

As a registered dental care professional, your registration will be in jeopardy if you break the law and put your patients at risk. The GDC provide advice and guidance about professional conduct. Advice can be found on their website. If you get into trouble with the police for even the most minor indiscretion, the fact will be reported to the GDC who may or may not take action against you. This includes motoring offences, cautions etc.

- *6.1. Justify the trust that your patients the public and your colleagues have in you, by always acting honestly and fairly.*

As a registered professional you are duty bound to act at all times in an honest and fair way. Doing otherwise will not only put your registration at risk but could also put you at risk of criminal proceedings.

- *6.3. Maintain appropriate standards of personal behaviour in all walks of life so that patients have confidence in you and the public have confidence in the dental profession.*

This means that should you do anything which puts either your own or the dental professional's reputation at risk you could be removed from the register of DCP. This includes any circumstances in which the police become involved i.e. public order, drunkenness, motoring offences. Then the GDC will be informed and you could be asked to explain yourself in front of the disciplinary committee.

Remember: If your name is removed from the register you cannot legally work as a dental nurse.

The *Standards for Dental Professionals* (2008) also gives guidelines on the treatment of patients under general anaesthetics or conscious sedation. There is a post qualification certificate available in conscious sedation. To find out more information about this course, contact the National Examination Board for Dental Nurses (NEBDN), in Fleetwood. They can provide a list of course providers, costs and course prospectus. You should refuse to assist a dentist in this type of treatment if you don't hold this certificate. A one day information session is not sufficient for working safely with patients undergoing this type of treatment.

## What are my obligations regarding equal opportunity?

- *2.3. Treat patients fairly and in line with the law. Promote equal opportunities for all patients, do not discriminate against patients or groups of patients because of their sex, age, race, ethnic origin, nationality, special needs or disability, sexuality, health, lifestyle, beliefs or other relevant consideration.*

The biggest impact this could have on your working practice is if you routinely take extra precautions when treating a patient who has a known infection or is a carrier of a blood borne infection. All patients attending for treatment must be treated equally. In terms of infection control and decontamination, all procedures must be the same to ensure the prevention of cross contamination and infection.

## What are my responsibilities to the patient to ensure they understand what their treatment involves?

- *2.4 Listen to patients and give them the information they need, in a way they can use, so that they can make decisions.*

This means that you should ensure that patients understand completely what they are being told. The information you give needs to be in a form that they can understand. This means not using jargon or technical terms. The patient must be fully aware of the treatment that is proposed and, where necessary, the full cost of the treatment. The patient must be able to

*Professional practice requirements and CPD*

make an informed decision and give consent from a basis of understanding.

## What are my responsisbilities regarding patient confidentiality?

- *3.1. Treat information about patients as confidential and only use it for the purposes for which it is given.*

This means that any information disclosed should not be discussed outside the working environment i.e. on the bus, in public areas of the practice or clinic, in a lift etc.

- *3.2. Prevent information from being accidentally revealed and prevent unauthorised access by keeping information secure at all times.*

This means not leaving patient notes lying around where other people can read them and ensuring that any electronic records are kept secure. This is also true of disclosing information to people on the telephone i.e. someone calling to see if a patient has attended for an appointment or enquiring about the treatment carried out. You cannot be sure who you are speaking to on the telephone or who may be listening. They may not be the person they say they are.

## What are my responsibilities to other members of the team?

- *4.1. Co-operate with other team members and colleagues and respect their role in caring for patients.*

Working in any type of dental institution has to be a team effort. No one person can do all the jobs involved. An efficient practice is one where every staff member knows their roles and responsibilities. This will lead to the patient receiving the best possible treatment in the best possible environment.

- *4.3. Communicate effectively and share your knowledge and skills*

93

> with other team members and colleagues as necessary in the interests of patients.

'A team is only as strong as its weakest member', is a well known saying and is particularly pertinent to dental teams. Most practice teams will include a trainee, either a nurse or a vocational trainee dentist, who may be the weakest member of the team as they lack knowledge and expertise. It is the responsibility of all the qualified team members to pass on their knowledge and skills and communicate to other members of the team so that everyone fully understands their role.

## What should I do if I feel that the patients are not being treated correctly?

> - *1.7. If you believe that patients might be at risk because of your health, behaviour or professional performance or that of a colleague or because of any aspect of the clinical environment, you should take action.*

This means that if someone you work with puts the wellbeing of patients at risk you must report it to the GDC. If you do not, and knowingly work in an unsafe way because of the actions of colleagues, then you will also be liable. This relates to anyone you work with: dentist, nursing colleague, hygienist, receptionist etc.

You have a responsibility to report any other registered professional who does not fully comply with the standards required of their professional registration. This has huge implications for not only you but also for every registered professional that you work with.

If you report a dentist, you could well have your employment terminated and find it difficult to obtain further employment. This provides you with a dilemma. If you do report the person, you could be out of work. But if you don't and a patient makes a complaint against the practice, you could be brought before the GDC Disciplinary Committee or Fitness to Practice Committees. It is for this reason that it is imperative that you have personal indemnity insurance and do not rely on a policy taken out by the practice owner which covers all staff. A policy that covers the whole practice may not provide sufficient protection to provide assistance in such an instance.

Since registration, all registered professionals are responsible for their actions and can be brought to account to the GDC. If your defence is that you knew things were not being done in a correct manner but were in fear of losing your job if you reported it, this argument will not protect you from possibly losing your registration and therefore, your job.

This is a difficult action to take and there are organisations that you can turn to for help and advice such as the Colleagues Defence Organisation, Professional Organisation or the GDC. Remember you may not want to 'whistle blow' on a colleague but would they worry about doing the same to you in a similar incident?

## What indemnity insurance do I need?

- *1.6. Make sure your patients are able to claim any compensation that they may be entitled to by making sure you are protected against claims at all times, including past periods of practice.*

Since the advent of compulsory registration in 2008, it has become possible for registered dental nurses to be sued by patients if they feel that they have not been treated correctly. Registered dental nurses are now responsible for their own actions and could be reported to the GDC who will take action either via the Disciplinary Committee or the Fitness to Practice Committee. Defending yourself in either hearing could cost many thousands of pounds and you would need the services of a barrister to represent you.

If the dentist you work for says that you are covered by their insurance, you should check carefully as it may not cover you for all eventualities. You should protect yourself by taking out an appropriate indemnity insurance policy and you should not rely solely on the cover given by a practicewide policy which covers everyone, it may not cover you sufficiently. If you work for your local personal dental service, in a NHS establishment or in a hospital, do not rely on 'Crown Indemnity', this will definitely not give sufficient cover if you are called to appear before either committee. The GDC do not state that this is compulsory but they strongly advise all registrants of whatever profession to be adequately covered by indemnity insurance.

Do not be lulled into a false sense of security, dental nurses have been called before the disciplinary committee and have been removed from the register. This means that they cannot work as a dental nurse.

When it comes to protecting your registration and ultimately your job and career, your insurance is vital but finding the right insurance is not so straight forward. There are many companies in this field and you must get all the information you can from all in the field and then make your choice as to whether or not it is sufficient. The GDC does give some guidance on its website (www.gdc-uk.org).

The BADN offers indemnity cover as part of their membership fee, but there are many dental defence organisations which can provide comprehensive information and advice. All these policies will cost money but the cheapest is not necessarily the best. What is not in question is the fact that you must have indemnity insurance.

## Why is indemnity insurance important for practice?

It is important to ensure that if an accident happens, the patient can claim and you are covered against that claim and defend yourself. If you are ultimately struck off the GDC register because of disciplinary action, then you cannot work, legally, as a dental nurse. Ultimately you will not be able to work, legally.

## What happens if I am not covered?

If you do not have sufficient indemnity insurance then, should an accident happen and the patient sues, you may not be able to properly defend yourself without legal advice. If you are referred to the Disciplinary Committee of the GDC then you will need a barrister to defend you and that is extremely costly. If you rely on the cover provided by your dentist's insurance you may not be fully covered. Should you lose your case then you run the risk of being struck off the register which will mean that you can no longer work as a dental nurse.

## What should I do if a claim is made against me?

If a claim is made against you then you should immediately contact your

*Professional practice requirements and CPD*

indemnity insurance provider to seek advice and help. If you believe you are covered by your dentist's insurance, you should contact the company and check just what cover you have and does it cover you for the claim if you are taken to the GDC? If you are unsure, then make enquiries from other providers and check which is going to be the best for you.

If you do not have indemnity insurance then you should seek advice from a solicitor.

## What are my obligations regarding continuing professional development (CPD)?

- *5.1. Recognise that your qualification for registration was the first stage in your professional education, develop and update your knowledge and skills throughout your working life.*

Your qualification is the start of your lifelong learning. The profession of dentistry never stands still. Someone somewhere is always researching new materials, procedures and techniques and it is important that everyone keeps up-to-date with all advances in dentistry. This will lead to improved job satisfaction, better team working and therefore improved treatment for your patients.

- *5.3. Find out about current best practice in the fields in which you work. Provide a good standard of care based on available up-to-date evidence and reliable guidance.*

This is also part of your lifelong learning. Providing the highest possible standards in all that you do must be the motto for everything you do. You should also be a role model for trainees within the practice.

The British Association of Dental Nurses (BADN) is a professional organisation solely concerned with looking after dental nurses. They produce a quarterly journal and hold an annual conference. They will provide advice to dental nurses who are members and membership includes indemnity insurance cover. They also have a local group network who organise evening seminars which provide CPD.

You can find latest information and keep up to date with changes to dental practice, materials and research by reading journals such as

*Dental Nursing Journal, Dental Practice, Vital* etc. You can also receive information from representatives from manufacturing companies and suppliers. They will often set up a training session to suit the practice and provide verifiable CPD for attendees.

Local post graduate deaneries will set up CPD courses and you should contact your local deanery to find out what they provide. These courses are usually held outside work hours and do usually incur a cost.

## How can I gain my Continuing Professional Development?

You have your basic qualification, congratulations. This must not be the end of your learning experience, you must carry on learning. To fulfil your GDC registration, you must complete 150 hours of CPD in a 5 year cycle, 50 hours of which must be verifiable. Verifiable means that the learning must be in the form of lectures, seminars or practical teaching which is accredited by the GDC and a certificate is awarded on completion. There are four core subjects that must be subject to CPD every year. These are:

- **Medical emergencies** including emergency drugs and Cardio-pulmonary Resuscitation (CPR) – 10 hours in every 5 year cycle.
- **Decontamination and disinfection** – 5 hours in every 5 year cycle.
- **Radiography and radiation protection** – 5 hours in every 5 year cycle.
- **Ethical and legal matters and complaints handling** – no set hours per cycle but recommended.

It is important that these subjects are studied every year and not all in just one year. They are important subjects for the safe running of the practice that you work in.

Non-verifiable CPD makes up the other 100 hours which is made up of learning you carry out by reading journals, watching videos etc. This learning will keep your knowledge up to date. In an ever changing profession, this is only the start you can achieve so much more and build a career in a progressive profession.

The practicalities of obtaining this learning may seem overwhelming but when broken down over the 5 year cycle, you only have to obtain 10 hours of verifiable CPD and 20 hours of non-verifiable CPD per year. Spread that over 12 months and that equates to just over 4 hours total each month.

Most seminars, workshops and lectures are for at least an hour and a visit from a representative to demonstrate new materials or equipment can easily be 2 hours. A team meeting in the practice can add a further 2 hours. If you help to update a practice policy or write such a policy on your own, this can be counted as non-verifiable CPD. If you attend a lecture, you can feedback to your colleagues and let them know what it was about, this can be counted as non-verifiable CPD.

When you have achieved this CPD you must compile it in the form of a portfolio, where you reference your CPD and provide evidence of the amount of time you have spent on each subject. Any certificates you obtain for attending a lecture, seminar etc should be kept and have your GDC registration number on it and the number of hours spent. Each year when you renew your registration you will be asked to submit how many hours CPD you have completed. Although this may not be audited each year, you may be audited at the end of the cycle and if your CPD does not meet with the standard, then you could put your registration at risk.

Nurses are only in the middle of their first cycle of CPD requirements. Dentists have had to collect CPD for some time and those who did not meet the CPD requirements were given a short time to obtain the missing amounts and those that did not were suspended from the register and hence were not allowed to practice. It is probable that a similar course of action will be taken with errant dental nurses.

This CPD should not be looked upon as a chore but more as an opportunity to interact with your colleagues, meet new friends and improve your knowledge and your skills to improve your job satisfaction.

There are many journals available for study, apart from the official journals of various professional sssociations such as the British Dental Association, British Society of Periodontology. British Endodontics Society, British Association of Dental Nurses, Infection Prevention Society. There is also publications such as the *Dental Nursing Journal, The Dentist, Dental Practice, Vital* etc. All these journals contain scientific articles, news of advances in research and updates in best practice. They also contain lists of courses that can be attended to accrue CPD and also courses that will lead to GDC approved extra responsibilities such as fluoride application, impression taking, advanced certificate in radiography, conscious sedation and special needs etc.

It is also advisable to register with your local post graduate deanery

*Dental Nurse Survival Guide*

who will arrange a series of lectures, workshops and seminars throughout the year at a small cost. They concentrate on arranging meetings that cover the core subjects.

You should be conscious that there are programmes on the television from time to time that can give CPD and keep an eye on the TV schedules.

Many dental nurses panicked when they first had to achieve CPD and enrolled for every lecture, seminar and course that was available and then realised that they had far more than they needed in the first year. They also realised that achieving the expected amount of hours was achievable without spending all their free time on it.

If you have any doubts, questions or concerns about CPD then consult the GDC website where more information can be found as well as proforma for the referencing of your CPD and advice on how to collect it. Remember that you must keep the evidence of your CPD for the full 5 years of the CPD cycle. If you do not keep it and cannot produce the evidence if asked, then it will be deemed to not exist. After the end of the 5 year cycle, you should keep all your evidence for a while because it may be some months before you are asked to produce your evidence and the people who are asked are picked at random.

## Should my employer provide my CPD?

It is your responsibility to complete your 150 hours of CPD in every 5 year cycle. If your employer allows you time off to attend seminars, courses, exhibitions etc so that you can obtain CPD hours, then you are very fortunate and you should take very opportunity that arises. If your employer does not give you time then there is nothing you can do other than to achieve your requirements in your own time and at your own expense.

It is possible to get verifiable CPD points from registered journals and online content and non-verifiable is relatively easily obtained by reading journals etc. It is possible that representatives from dental suppliers will come into the practice to give training which can be used for verifiable CPD. Dentists also have to complete CPD and many courses organised for them have DCP parts added to them, to encourage dentists to take their team to learn at the same time.

It is to the dentist's advantage to encourage their staff to take time to complete their CPD and to report back to team meetings to share what they have learned. If your dentist returns from a seminar or exhibition with a new piece of equipment then he must make sure you understand its uses, purpose and how it is decontaminated and sterilised and maintained. It's pointless spending money on new kit if it either stays in a cupboard because no-one knows how to use it or it is broken at its first use because of misunderstandings with decontamination etc.

## What further training can I do to improve my career?

Compulsory registration has brought new opportunities for dental nurses. For some years post qualification certificates have been available, namely:

- Treating patients under conscious sedation
- Oral health education
- Radiography.

All these courses are accredited by the NEBDN and are recognised qualifications of specialist knowledge. In some circumstances they can lead to increased pay but they should always give increased job satisfaction and improved treatment for your patients.

Since registration the number of certificated courses has increased and will continue to increase over the coming years. New courses include:

- Special needs nursing
- Orthodontic specialist nursing
- Impression taking.

The list will continue to grow to encompass other aspects of the GDC's *Scope of Practice for Dental Nurses*.

## What career paths are available for dental nurses?

It is a cliché but in dental nursing terms, 'The world is your oyster'. There is now the potential to make dental nursing a true career with a very real chance of promotion and advancement.

Apart from specialising in different aspects of practical chair–side dental nursing there are opportunities to gain extra qualifications in teaching to become a tutor. There are possibilities to take on extra responsibilities as a senior dental nurse or a practice manager. There are qualifications available for practice managers and there is now a foundation degree available for dental nurses which would open up the route to higher management. You should study the university or college prospectuses to obtain information about suitable courses. The post graduate deanery may also have information about such courses.

There are positions within the salaried services, dental hospitals, personal dental services etc. at a higher management level. These are known as Dental Nurse Managers or Principal Dental Nurses. These posts are purely administrative and usually offer no chair-side nursing. Post holders are expected to manage large numbers of staff and introduce new policies and procedures and instigate new working practices. They are usually responsible for managing or supervising the management of a dental nurse training scheme.

As a career, dental nursing can take you as far as you wish. If what you want is a fulfilling career at the chair-side without the responsibilities of management, then you can follow that path and enjoy the patient contact. If you want responsibility that includes managing staff, although with less chair-side patient contact, then you can also follow that path. If you want to specialise in one aspect of dental nursing, then that path is open to you by enrolling on an accredited post qualification course in that speciality.

It really is up to you but no-one will do the research for available course for you, you really have to make the effort yourself. Whichever paths you choose, dental nursing can fulfil all your ambitions.

## Should my practice principal keep my GDC registration certificate?

The answer is most definitely NO. Your GDC certificate is your property and more importantly, it is the only tangible proof you have that you are registered. It is possible to check your registration on the GDC website but not all employers will want to do that and you need to be able to give them the practical evidence of your registration. If your employer needs to keep proof of your registration, which they almost certainly will, then they should take a photocopy and sign it to certify it.

## Should my employer employ qualified nurses who are not registered?

Your employer's ethics must be called into question if they are willing to consider employing unregistered nurses and call them dental nurses, without registering them on an accredited training scheme.

It is illegal for anyone to be employed as a dental nurse if they are not registered on the GDC register and you should report the dentist to the GDC if they do employ such unregistered staff. The same goes for any laboratory technician who is not registered.

## References

General Dental Council (2008) *Standards for Dental Professionals*
General Dental Council (2008) *Guidance for Registrants*
General Dental Council (2008) *Patient Confidentiality Booklet*
General Dental Council (2008) *Team Working Booklet*
General Dental Council (2008) *Complaints Handling Booklet*
General Dental Council (2008) *Raising Concerns Booklet*
General Dental Council (2008) *Management Responsibility Booklet*
General Dental Council (2008) *Scope of Practice for Dental Nurses*
The General Dental Council – www.GDC-UK.org

# CHAPTER 9

# The dental practice team and culture

- **Who is in the team?**
- **What role does the receptionist play in the team?**
- **What role does the dental nurse play in the team?**
- **What role does the dentist play in the team?**
- **What role does the hygienist play in the team?**
- **What role does the practice manager play in the team?**
- **What role do the cleaners play in the team?**
- **What role do the external laboratory staff play in the team?**
- **What is the style of the establishment that you work in?**

Wherever you work within the dental nursing profession, be it in general dental practice, dental hospital or personal dental service, you will be working as part of a team. It is imperative that all staff working in the institution are a team, if you cannot work as a team you cannot deliver high quality services to your patients.

## Who is in the team?

The team consists of every person working in the establishment. In a large dental hospital, this will be divided up into departments but all the departments must work as a team to achieve the goals and objectives of the organisation.

To achieve the highest standard of care for your patients, everyone who works in your practice must be part of the team delivering the care from the moment they arrive at the practice to the moment they leave and includes all the time they are in the building. Members of the team include:
- The Receptionist.
- The Dental Nurse.
- The Dentist.

- The Hygienist.
- The Practice Manager.
- The Cleaners.
- Staff outside laboratories.

All these differing professions must work in harmony to provide the highest possible standard of patient care, as well as keeping the other team members motivated and working to the best of their ability and enjoying their jobs and roles. A happy workforce or team will ensure a high quality patient experience.

## What role does the receptionist play in the team?

The receptionist is the first person that the patient meets. It is vital that your receptionist welcomes the patient. They must present a caring attitude and understand that a patient is most likely nervous and possibly very apprehensive. The receptionist needs to be able to efficiently deal with appointment requests and may also have to deal with the clerical duties involved with payments. They must be aware of how to deal with difficult situations which may arise from irate patients who have been kept waiting or were not able to be given an appointment when they wanted one.

Depending on clerical arrangements within the practice, they may need to have treatment notes available for the dentist at the time the patient is treated.

They are the first point of contact and must demonstrate the practice's caring attitude and high standards of care towards the patient. They must also be trained in the practice's policies and procedures on how to deal with emergencies. Emergencies can arise in the waiting room as well as in the treatment room. The waiting area is their 'domain' and it is their responsibility to keep tidy during the day and it should be somewhere that they can take a pride in.

## What role does the dental nurse play in the team?

The dental nurse is, arguably, the most important person in the whole team.

You must present the caring face of the practice. It is you that the patient will turn to for comfort, support and explanation when they are being treated. The apprehensive or nervous patient will need to know that the nurse is 'there for them'. The dentist can cause them pain and is the person they are afraid of; the nurse is there to look after them and make the dental experience as tolerable as possible.

You must prepare everything the dentist needs and be prepared to change everything at a moment's notice if the dentist changes his/her treatment plans. You must be responsible for ensuring effective infection prevention and control within the treatment area, organising and arranging the cleanliness of the treatment area and the decontamination and sterilisation of contaminated instruments and equipment. You will have a large responsibility for ensuring that aspects of *Health Technical Memorandum 01-05 Decontamination in Dental Practice*, (HTM 01-05) (DoH 2008) are complied with. You will not have overall responsibility, that lies with the dentist, but they will rely on you to ensure high standards of compliance within your sphere of knowledge. You are also responsible for daily checks for safety of certain equipment before patients are treated. See Chapter 3 for more details about daily practices and responsibilities.

There must be good communication between you and the receptionist to ensure patients are not kept waiting. If this is unavoidable, then you must communicate the reasons to the receptionist to relate to the patient.

You must also communicate well with your patients to ensure their understanding of what is happening so that they can give informed consent to treatment. You must be able to make sure they understand without using jargon or technical terms. You must also be able to communicate the patient's concerns and worries to the dentist.

You must work effectively and efficiently to ensure the patient's treatment is carried out with the minimum of fuss and as smoothly as possible. Not only will this ensure a good patient experience but also that the dentist can treat as many patients to a high standard to meet financial targets. This must not, however, be your driving force. Your driving force must be high levels of treatment and good patient experience to ensure they return to complete their treatment and also, if asked, they will recommend your practice to other potential patients.

## What role does the dentist play in the team?

The dentist actually carries out the dental treatment required and sets the standards that other team members will work to.

The dentist sets the tone for how the practice is run. They will influence whether the practice is run to simply make as much profit as possible, irrespective of the quality of care, or whether the patient experience is paramount.

The dentist owns the practice or is an associate of the owner. Through team meetings they will ensure that the practice is run efficiently, that all paperwork, reports, legal requirements etc are met. They must oversee that all members of the team work together to achieve the goals that they are set. They must be approachable, willing to explain fully what they require but must also be willing to take action if team members underperform and ensure that such a team member receives the extra support they require. The dentist must also ensure that new staff or team members are thoroughly trained in the procedures of the practice.

The dentist sets the ethos for the work carried out in the practice.

## What role does the hygienist play in the team?

The hygienist carries out specific types of treatment as prescribed by the dentist. The treatment they carry out must add to the patient experience in a positive way.

They can spot problems and refer patients back to the dentist. They must communicate effectively with the nurse and receptionist to ensure the highest possible standard of patient care. The hygienist must be involved in planning changes, new policies and procedures and any other aspect of ensuring the practice works efficiently to achieve good patient care and a continuing full appointment book.

## What role does the practice manager play in the team?

The practice manager must 'manage' the practice. This will involve the administration and clerical work, contracts and required official documents, ordering stock, materials, organising ancillary staff etc.

All this must be done with the other team members; although the practice manager must take responsibility for aspects of the management, they cannot do all of it on their own. They must have the support and co-operation of all the other team members. There must be a close working

*The dental practice team and culture*

relationship so that problems can be recognised, investigated and resolved as quickly as possible to ensure the continuing smooth running of the practice.

Practice managers must also be involved in decision making and must be prepared to instigate change for the good of the practice. Training is available for practice managers and ongoing updating and revision courses should be identified and attended.

## What role do the cleaners and ancillary staff play in the team?

The public areas of the practice, such as the waiting area, reception area, toilets, staff room, office, treatment area floor etc must be regularly and effectively cleaned and must always be tidy, with old magazines disposed of, toys kept clean and tidy. These areas show the practice's public face and will make the first impression to new and existing patients.

They must feel part of the team and be involved and valued in the practice. If the cleaners feel part of the team and valued, they will want to give a good standard of service and take a pride in their work.

## What role do the external laboratory staff play?

There must be good communication between outside laboratories and the practice to ensure full understanding of what is required by the laboratory in the form of documentation, decontamination etc.

This must be a two way communication and any concerns raised by either establishment should be rapidly and efficiently addressed. It is imperative that the practice sends good quality impressions and instruction so that the laboratory can produce high quality prostheses, direct and indirect restorations.

## What is the style of the establishment that you work in?

When you first join a practice or other establishment, you need to find out what is expected of the team. You need to find out what drives the ethos of the establishment:

1. Are the patients' just the way of earning more money?

Or

2. Is maintaining the highest standard of patient care the only important consideration?

If the patient is just viewed as a way of maximising earnings then the quality of the treatment may not be the most important consideration. It will be more important to see as many patients as possible and do the most costly types of treatment; costly that is, to the patient, but not to the dentist. Patients who require time consuming treatment will be referred to specialist care. You may be expected to use the cheapest possible materials, PPE and decontamination and sterilisation materials and techniques. This could bring the establishment into conflict with monitoring and statutory bodies. Practices are being inspected by the Care Quality Commission (CQC) and must ultimately be registered with them to continue practicing. If standards are not of an acceptable level then the practice could be closed down.

If, on the other hand, the treatment provided to the patient is of the paramount importance and although cost cannot be ignored, it is not the driving force, then decisions made in the practice will be in the best interests of the patient. They will be given time to ask questions. Patients will only be referred to a specialist if the treatment required can only be carried out by those specialists. The practice will possibly train vocational trainees and employ trainee dental nurses. Most importantly, they will enrol those trainee nurses on an accredited training course. Not only that, they will give all trainees all the support that they can. Materials used, PPE used and decontamination and sterilisation materials and techniques will be the best that can be achieved in the situation of the practice.

Practices, as well as other establishments, must be financially stable but must also provide the highest level of treatment as well as treating all the staff in the team as being important. Everyone should be working towards the common goal of high standards of treatment carried out by a highly skilled and motivated team in a safe and caring environment.

## References

Department of Health (2008) *Health Technical Memorandum 01-05 Decontamination in Dental Practice*

# Index

## A

adrenal insufficiency 9, 17
AIDS 42
anaphylaxis 8, 10–11
angina 8, 11
aspiration 16
asthma 8, 9–10
automated external defibrillator 3
avulsed teeth, treatment of 21

## B

bad news
  offering the patient support 83–84
  responsibility for giving 83
biopsy appointments 81
bridges 68

## C

children, treatment of 72–73
choking 16
claims, against dental nurses 97
cleaning of PPE 45
complaints handling, CPD requirements for 98
computerised record keeping 65
CPD
  dental nurse's obligations for 97–98
  employers' responsibility for 100
Control of Substances Hazardous to Health 1988 (COSHH) 41
cross infection 37–42
crowns 68

## D

decontamination 29–30
  CPD requirements 98
  of PPE 45
  procedures 31–34
dental

emergencies 19–22
nurse
  responsibilities of 27–28, 92–94
  career paths 102
  principles of practice for 90
denture appointments 69
disinfection, CPD requirements 98

## E

electrocardiograms (ECG) 4
endodontic appointments 70
Environmental Protection Act (1990) 42
epileptic seizures 9, 12–13
equal opportunities 92
ethical matters, CPD requirements 98
ethics, employers' 103
extractions 76–77
extra-oral radiographs 55
eye protection 45

## F

face masks 44
facial trauma, treatment of 20
fillings 67

## G

GDC registration certificate 102
gloves 44

## H

hand
  hygiene 48
  washing 46, 47
Health and Safety at Work Act 1974 41
hepatitis B 42
HIV 42
hygiene, hand/personal 48
hypoglycaemia 14
hypoglycaemic attack 8

111

*Index*

# I

implant appointments 79–80
indemnity insurance 95, 96
infections, protection against 42
insurance
  needs of dental nurses 95
intra-oral radiographs, processing of 56
Ionising Radiation Regulations 52, 53

# L

legal matters, CPD requirements for 98

# M

Management of Health and Safety at Work Regulations 1999 41
materials
  impression 64
  powder and liquid 64
  two paste 65
medical emergency
  CPD requirements 98
  drugs and equipment 4–5
  tips on avoiding 5–6
  what to do in 3–4, 6–7
myocardial infarction 9, 12

# N

newly qualified dental nurse
  responsibilities of 27–28
new patient assessment 66
nurse's role during treatment 61–62

# O

onlay 68
orthodontic appointments 71

# P

paperwork 65
patients
  dealing with difficult 85–86
  assessment 66
  confidentiality 93

periodontal appointments 73–74, 80
personal hygiene 48
personal protective equipment (PPE) 43, 44
post qualification certificates 101
principles of dental practice 90
pulse oximeter 3

# R

radiographs
  assisting with 2
  dealing with processing chemicals 57
  processing of 56, 57
  qualification for taking 51
  training to perform 51
radiography
  CPD requirements 54, 98
  digital 58–59
  infection prevention and control measures 59–60
  laws and rules concerning 52–53
review appointments 78–79

# S

sedation 75
sharps injury 49
Standard Precautions 38–39, 43
Standards for Dental Professionals 90, 90–92
sterilisation of PPE 45
supervision during training 25
surgical procedures 77–78
suture removal 78–79
swelling, treatment of 22
syncope 8, 15, 16

# T

telephone queries 85
treatment records
  computerised 65

# U

uniform protection 45